AF531590

PERSPECTIVES OF HEALTH EDUCATION

PERSPECTIVES OF HEALTH EDUCATION

PREGNANCY AND CHILD BIRTH

VOL. 2

MARY RALF

ANMOL PUBLICATIONS PVT. LTD.
NEW DELHI-110 002 (INDIA)

ANMOL PUBLICATIONS PVT. LTD.
4374/4B, Ansari Road, Daryaganj
New Delhi-110 002

Perspectives of Health Education : Pregnancy and Child Birth

First Edition 1998
ISBN 81-7488-932-9 (Set)

PRINTED IN INDIA

Published by J. L. Kumar for Anmol Publications Pvt. Ltd., New Delhi-110 002 and Printed at Tarun Offset Printers, Delhi.

Contents

17

Woman of the Century

Had Mike Wallace actually been interested in reporting on developments in family planning, there was quite a bit to say. In the waning years of the 1950s, basic assumptions that had long constrained movement activists were finally being altered in a manner that would allow for dramatic gains during the following two decades.

The big news, of course, was scientific. Planned Parenthood's own clinical experience had long demonstrated the limitations of the diaphragm and jelly and provided the most convincing rationale of all for better technology, if birth control was to be truly democratized. It was hardly surprising, therefore, when the preliminary findings on the pill published by Gregory Pincus and John Rock in 1956 led immediately to expanded field trials. Within a year, the Population Council had agreed to joint meetings with the International Planned Parenthood Federation to discuss technology and was directly supporting field research on a small sample of pill takers in Los Angeles. And a larger experiment was begun in Puerto Rico, under the direction of a local public health physician by the name of Edris Rice-Wray, whom Pincus had met while giving a lecture in San Juan.

As a legacy of Ernest Gruening's and Clarence Gamble's quiet cooperation during the Depression, the Puerto Rican legislature had legalized birth control in 1937, over the strident objections of the Catholic Church. Sixty-three family planning clinics remained in operation on the island, one of them in a housing project for indigent families where Dr. Rice-Wray worked. A tradition of sexual modesty and the absence of reliable methods prevented the island's women from practicing conventional contraception effectively, however, and sterilization had instead become their contraceptive of choice. Promoted by private physicians eager for the business and inadvertently by Catholic pastoral letters condemning it, sterilization was not just reliable but had the distinct advantage of requiring only a one-time absolution in the confessional. In a pattern that the United States mainland would begin to replicate in the 1970s, one third of all women ages twenty to forty-nine were having the operation. Yet the Puerto Rican birthrate still remained twice as high as the United States national average.

Under these circumstances Dr. Rice-Wray had no trouble finding recruits for her pill research and no compunction about recommending that they take a risk on experimental medication. In one year she collected data for several hundred patients, aggregating forty-seven years of pill-taking, without a single pregnancy. Problems with side effects such as nausea, fluid retention, and dizziness caused a quarter of the original sample to drop out, but eager substitutes were found, and experiments with placebos then demonstrated that at least some of these reactions were psychological, while the administration of the actual medication in lower dosages resolved even more problems, with still no effect on contraceptive reliability.

Anxious officials in the local public health ministry, nevertheless, put a stop to the research when they learned of it, and Dr. Rice-Wray left the country for a position in Mexico. A second field trial was then arranged privately in the village of Humacao as the result of a proposal by Clarence Gamble to Dr. Adaline Pendleton Satterthwaite, a Quaker medical missionary there. Having spent years delivering babies and then sterilizing desperately poor women, she too had no trouble defending her work on humanitarian grounds and wound up providing a fourth of the case histories on which Gregory Pincus would base his successful argument for the safety and effectiveness of Enovid before the United States Food and Drug Administration three years later.

Physicians and policymakers in the continental United States were, at first, considerably more cautious. During the summer of 1957, Planned Parenthood officials in New York issued a tentative statement of support for the Pincus-Rock studies in Brookline, but admonished enthusiasts who were already proclaiming the dawn of a new era that it was still much too soon to regard the medication as safe. Dr. Carl Hartman, then chairman of the organization's medical committee, expressed many reservations about the possible consequences of altering the body's natural hormonal chemistry and predicted a fifteen-to-twenty-year period before the drug's safety could be assured. (This prompted Margaret to pencil in the comment on her copy of the statement that he was simply "jealous.") In fact, Planned Parenthood would take close to two years after FDA approval before authorizing the pill's use by its affiliates, during which time Searle and Ortho Pharmaceuticals, its first major competitor, substantially reduced the drug's progestin and estrogen content, further diminishing reported side effects and enhancing safety.

Private physicians who had never liked the diaphragm, because prescribing it was neither medically challenging nor terribly remunerative, turned out to be a good deal more enthusiastic about the pill and within five years it became the most popular contraceptive in America, used by 29 percent of married, non-Catholic women under the age of forty-five and by more than half of all women with a college education. It would soon revolutionize contraceptive practice among Catholics as well. Close to 50 million women around the world would be taking oral contraceptives by the 1970s, a population more than adequate to establish their reliability and safety for women of normal health—outside a small and readily identifiable group of high-risk users. Sixty million use it today. Periodic alarms about the relationship of the pill to embolisms, cancers, and other serious complications have been sounded, but never substantiated in large enough numbers to dissuade use. From a medical standpoint, the potent drug, whose actual physiological effects to this day remain poorly understood, has proved remarkably benign, even as women have continued to question the wisdom of taking it over long periods of time.

The demographic consequences of oral contraception have also been substantial, though never enough so to satisfy population planners. The pill's early and rapid success did demonstrate the motivation of large numbers of women, across a broad spectrum of classes, creeds and cultures, and helped undermine prevailing assumptions about who would use contraception and who would not. But because it remained a relatively costly medication, requiring prescription by a doctor and individual daily administration, it never lived up to the hopes of its early patrons. International population professionals have continued to look for an inexpensive technology that does not depend on the regular cooperation of the people using it—something on the order of the inoculations against epidemic disease that have more successfully revolutionized maternal and child health around the world.

These inherent liabilities were, in fact, recognized from the start. In 1957, while field trials on the pill were still underway, officials at the Population Council continued to despair over the prospects for ever bringing about meaningful change through voluntary family planning initiatives. A long-term experiment with conventional barrier and chemical methods of contraception in Khanna, a rural district of India, was resulting in poor compliance and negligible changes in fertility. And even in the United States, where knowledge of contraception was nearly universal, and its use controversial only among a few groups, national fertility surveys were still uncovering substantial numbers of unwanted births. Accidental, unplanned pregnancies in and out of marriage remained a problem of statistical significance, especially among the poor, who appeared to have more difficulty anticipating the need for contraception, and less access to pharmacies or health care services that could provide it.

In 1958, the Population Council decided to invest in the development of a contraceptive device that could be left in place for a long period of time. Alan F. Guttmacher, M.D., then chief of obstetrics at Mt. Sinai Hospital in New York, and a member of the council's medical advisory board, recommended the support of preliminary research by Lazar Margulies, a German-trained physician on his staff, who was experimenting with a variation on the Grafenberg ring that Margaret had promoted years earlier and then been pressured to reject. The new intrauterine device substituted a pliant plastic material for the metal components that had always been difficult to insert and more likely to cause uterine punctures and infection. The once controversy-shy organization then contracted with Christopher Tietze, M.D., another German emigre who had become the protege of Robert Dickinson and had continued working on his own with a shoestring budget at the National Committee on Maternal Health following Dickinson's death. During the early 1960s several million dollars would be channeled through Tietze for the refinement, testing, and evaluation of various intrauterine devices. And the organization would reserve to itself the international marketing rights for a loop-shaped apparatus developed by the Buffalo physician Jack Lippes, that gained the highest rate of acceptance and caused the fewest side effects. By 1967, when the success of the pill had degitimized active intervention in family planning on a broad international scale, the Population Council would incorporate this research and technical assistance capacity as its own Bio-Medical division, where further testing and refinement of various IUDs, injectable contraceptives, and other experimental medications have continued.

IUDs were widely distributed in the 1970s and 1980s, but their use has declined substantially in recent years as a result of concerns about safety. IUDs have been associated with an increased risk of pelvic inflammatory disease, which, if left untreated, can cause sterility. The fear of malpractice liability has left many physicians in the United States unwilling to insert the devices, and they are also less frequently recommended anymore for use in countries where adequate follow-up medical care is not available to women. More successful in recent years has been the Population Council's investment in research on subdermal contraceptive implants that slowly release an ovulation inhibiting synthetic hormone containing progestin, and can remain in place for up to five years. Close to a million women in the rest of the world are currently using this procedure, and it has recently been approved for use in the United States by the Food and Drug Administration.

In the United States and many other countries, however, barrier contraceptives are still widely employed, sterilization remains a preferred option of married women who have completed their desired childbearing, and legal abortion is a widely utilized backup. This is likely to remain the case, so long as all artificial methods pose the risk of any side effects or more serious complications. As a result, the primary objectives of family planning policymakers today must be to promote additional research to ensure that existing services are tailored to the individual needs of women in disparate cultures and circumstances.

Political barriers to change were also eroding in the late 1950s. As Margaret had long complained, Planned Parenthood, after rejecting her own flamboyant, confrontational tactics, never formulated a coherent strategy for combating, or even neutralizing, the power of Catholic opposition to family planning and instead more or less accommodated to its marginal political and legal stature in this country.

Something of a turning point, however, came in 1955 when Agnes Meyer of Washington admonished new recruits to the organization to be less cowardly and encouraged them to articulate a positive vision in opposition to Catholic absolutism, thus demonstrating that they could no longer be intimidated.

The ideal circumstances for putting this advice into practice developed several years later, when a doctor in a municipal hospital in Brooklyn found that he could not get permission from New York city's health commissioner to fit a diabetic patient with a diaphragm. Hospital administrators and city officials sensitive to New York's large and powerful Catholic constituency had never challenged the unwritten but widely acknowledged policy that kept contraceptives out of publicly assisted health clinics, despite the legal protection state law provided birth control when prescribed for medical reasons. Indigent women could only find medical birth control through a handful of Planned Parenthood facilities and clinics in voluntary hospitals or settlement houses.

Working behind the scenes, Planned Parenthood staff in New York, under the direction of Frederick Jaffe, then a young and savvy public relations specialist, assembled a broad coalition of support from non-Catholic medical, social, and religious institutions. They also brought the situation to the attention of the local press, where it received extensive coverage, especially from Joseph Kahn, a crusading investigative reporter for the *New York Post,* who helped frame the issue as a matter of freedom of information, medical discretion, and religious tyranny. After months of concreted lobbying, the policy was overturned with the quiet acquiescence of Democratic Mayor Robert Wagner, Jr., though he remained neutral in public. Contraceptive services were subsequently incorporated into postpartum clinics in the city's three largest municipal hospitals, though only physicians, of course, not social workers or other non-medical personnel, could legally give information.

The New York city confrontation raised popular awareness of the substantial political constraints on birth control in this country. Editorial opinion was nearly unanimous in its approval of government's taking a more assertive role and gave Planned Parenthood professionals the courage to assist similar confrontations elsewhere. The victory also exposed emerging divisions of opinion within the Catholic Church itself. "It should be clear," suggested an article in *Commonweal*, by then considerably more liberal editorially than it had been in the past, "that there are many sound and compelling reasons why Catholics should not generally strive for legislation and directives which clash with the beliefs of a large portion of society...they almost inevitably strengthen in the minds of non-Catholics the already present worries about Catholic power." Two years later a Planned Parenthood poll of lay Catholics would establish that more than half believed public officials should respect freedom of religious belief in all medical institutions. An editorial in *The Pilot,* the publication of the Boston Archidiocese, then acknowledged that although Catholic principles remain constant, "the social, political, economic, legal and cultural context in which these principles are applied is itself in flux and they must be applied differently." No longer would the church be able to present itself as a monolith, absolutely resistant to change.

Margaret was in Tucson during the many months of the New York City encounter, preoccupied by the prosaic task of keeping herself alive. Her only participation was a telephone interview in which she called the city policy "disgraceful." she was no longer well enough to remain more than intermittently active. An increasingly constricted flow of blood to her weakened heart muscle was causing more frequent paroxysms of chest pain, and when stricken she required oxygen and extended rest. A New York specialist advised surgery, but her own doctors though that an open-heart procedure was too risky for a patient of her condition and age.

She was absorbed as well in something of a personal obsession that she blew way out of proportion—the question of who would replace her as president of the International Planned Parenthood Federation. The obvious candidates were Lady Rama Rau of India, who had for a time already shared the title with Margaret, and Elise Ottensen-Jensen of Sweden, who had brought considerable distinction upon herself as the conduit through which her government became the first Western nation to assist family planning programs in the developing world through a joint program with the government of Ceylon. With the United States and the United Nations still uninvolved, the agenda for a well-run and ambitious voluntary organization was pressing. The job would demand strong administrative skills and special sensitivity to the nuances of international diplomacy. On both grounds each candidate had liabilities acknowledged by many of Margaret's correspondents, yet her own reservations were scarcely rational. No one seemed to please her, and other women were especially threatening. Mrs. Rama Rau was too nationally minded, Mrs. Ottesen-Jensen, too temperamental. Fearful of finally having to yield her own authority completely, she promoted the candidacy of her long-time loyal lieutenant, Dr. Abraham Stone, but he died unexpectedly of a heart attack in 1959, and with international attention focused on India's population explosion, first Rama Rau and later Ottesen-Jensen got the job.

Margaret also insisted on attending the Sixth International Conference on Planned Parenthood in New Delhi in February of 1959, though her doctors and her family strongly advised her not to go. Grace Sternberg, a friend and Planned Parenthood volunteer from Tucson, agreed to act as travel companion and watched over an extremely frail patient who resolutely made her way from Los Angeles to Honolulu, Tokyo, Hong Kong, and Bangkok, complaining at each stop that she could not tolerate the fact that everyone thought she was dying, even as she wearily retreated from each festivity tendered in her honor.

Ample reward for her determination and stamina came when Prime Minister Nehru warmly welcomed Margaret to the meetings in New Delhi on February 14, 1959, and then cautiously ushered her on his arm to the podium as the 750 delegates who had assembled from twenty-eight nations put aside their differences to cheer the moving sight. Nehru pledged $10 million in public health funds for family planning, earning Margaret's praise as the world's greatest living statesman, along with a trenchant warning that he be careful to send doctors into the villages who were sympathetic to the "shy, simple woman who comes to them, asking for information as to how to space her pregnancies and how to take care of the children that she has already borne." It was a final opportunity to reiterate her view that how an individual woman perceives her own self-interest may be as important to her decisions about fertility as larger economic and social conditions. Stories and photographs ran in major newspapers and news magazines throughout the world, and Margaret was given the honor of being named president emeritus of IPPF.

The following day Gregory Pincus dedicated his historic report on field trials with oral contraception to Margaret as "the product of her pioneering resoluteness," but by then she was too weak to leave her hotel room and celebrated quietly with old friends over a favorite meal of champagne and chicken sandwiches. They presented her with a two-volume testimonial, entitled "Our M.S.," filled with the often poignant, personal reminiscences that have appeared throughout this book, and dedicated to the woman who "blazed a trail through the Jungle of Man's prejudice and Ignorance and Stupidity." The surprisingly strident tone o the collection was established by Blanche Ames of Boston, the first of more than a hundred contributors listed alphabetically, who observed acidly that monuments had been erected to the deeds of men since the time of the pyramids, but rarely was the work of a woman ever honored.

Yet even as Margaret's contemporaries tried to establish her place among history's foremost emancipation of women a newly empowered generation of activists was questioning the fundamental wisdom of her approach to family planning for the very reason that it enlisted women as clients and talked in terms of their self-interest. Dudley Kirk, a demographer on the Population Council staff, reminded his audience at New Delhi that "male" methods of contraception, such as the condom and coitus interruptus (as though neither required female participation) had actually been responsible for the great demographic revolutions of the West, and he advocated a policy for India that placed priority on these simple techniques rather than on expensive medical ones requiring individualized instruction. A proponent of sending convoys of helicopters laden with condoms into rural villages, Kirk was glad to observe the evolution of Planned Parenthood away from "emphasis on family limitation as primarily an interest and responsibility of women," he said, "toward emphasis on the value and indeed the necessity of joint responsibility in family planning."

Indeed the view that a "feminist bias" was subverting family planning programs in the developing world, where a medical-clinical approach to the problem was believed to be simply too expensive and likely to fail, would continue to inform the thinking of demographers and policy makers, even as new contraceptive methods for women revolutionized the field. In 1961, Katherine McCormick sadly admitted to Margaret in the last surviving letters between them that no one any longer believed that the pill was the answer to overpopulation. Her letter also said that Gregory Pincus was experimenting with injectable contraceptives but correctly predicted that effective inoculations would take years to develop. Meanwhile, programs offering economic incentives for male sterilization would probably be necessary in places like India, where the Nehru government was already supporting policies that have since engendered widespread controversy and been widely repudiated.

Since 1965, however, the rate of population growth has unexpectedly slowed in almost all countries in the world outside Africa, even as absolute numbers continue to grow precipitously everywhere but in a handful of developed nations. Most baffling, however, have been the extreme cultural variations in reproductive behavior and in the success of organized family planning initiatives. Efforts to understanding these patterns, and to analyse alternative strategies for intervention, are finally reawakening interest in the relationship between fertility and the status of women. Contemporary population policy-makers are more inclined to concede Margaret's insistent view that women are inherently better motivated to limit their fertility and should be identified as primary agents of change. Programs seem to work best, moreover, when contraception is offered as part of a larger package of maternal and infant health care reforms delivered under paramedical auspices, just as she always intended. Prodded by contemporary feminists in the field, population planners are finally investing in the overall health and welfare of women, because it has been demonstrated that to do so reduces birthrates most effectively.

Margaret returned from New Delhi in a wheelchair, a rather pathetic sight in Grace Sternberg's memory, except that she good-naturedly wore a straw hat purchased in Honolulu, which was adorned by a chicken whose wings flapped up and down when she pressed air through a bulb. Within months, however, she was feeling strong enough to fly back to Tokyo to meet with the Prime Minister and receive a key to the city from its governor. Accompanied by her teenaged granddaughters and several of their friends, she basked in an official recognition and esteem that had long been denied her at home. But the trip was a struggle, and she confided to Mary Lasker, who graciously underwrote its costs, that "I pray I will be well enough to do all that is expected of me."

The young girls, meanwhile, were entertained in memorable Japanese style by Sumiko Ohmori, who had married since her visit to Tucson and was anxious to return Margaret's gracious hospitality. Young Margaret and Nancy Sanger were astonished to find that, in Japan, not only family planning activists, but even taxi drivers had heard of their grandmother.

This would turn out to be Margaret's last trip abroad, and just how much it meant to her is apparent not only in her enthusiastic reports to Mrs. Lasker, but in a touching notation in the deteriorated handwriting of Margaret's old age, which remains on a scrap of paper included in the archive at Smith College. It records the wish that she be buried next to Noah in the family plot on the grounds of Willowlake, but only after her heart had been removed for entombment in Japan, the one government in the world that ever granted her a public honor.

Though birth control remained a politically sensitive issue at home, Margaret came back to a country suddenly paying attention. In response to pressure from Democrats on the powerful Senate Foreign Relations Committee, President Dwight David Eisenhower had appointed a special committee to assess his administration's policies on foreign military and economic aid. The ten-member panel of men who had all served previously in high-ranking government positions was chaired by Gen. William H. Draper, an investment banker and former army commander who had supervised postwar economic recovery programs in Europe. Prompted by a telegram from the ever-resolute population watchdog Hugh Moore—and given explicit authorization to do so from Eisenhower himself—Draper placed world population growth on the committee's agenda. There was considerable rumbling from his staff about potentially explosive political consequences and particular resistance from one especially anxious Catholic member of the panel. But while Margaret herself was still out of the country, Draper decided to recommend that the United States government should, on request, assist foreign governments receiving our economic aid in formulating plans to deal with population growth and with maternal and child welfare problems.

The report's release in July of 1959 received extensive press coverage and an immediate, but reasonably restrained, response from the National Catholic Welfare Conference branding its birth control recommendations "not only immoral (but) also a counsel of defeatism and despair." Popular interest in the issue built steadily in the months following, however, especially after CBS News in November ran a prime-time documentary on conditions of rural poverty and population growth in India, which would air twice and be seen by an estimated audience of more than 18 million Americans.

At meetings in Washington later that month, the American Catholic hierarchy then released a considerably more vituperative statement, attacking public discussion of the "population explosion" as nothing more than a "smoke screen behind which a moral evil will be foisted on the public" and denouncing efforts to build support for the use of public funds for artificial contraception. The church instead urged great efforts to feed and uplift "backward peoples around the world," and in pledging to work actively against population control programs, provoked the immediate condemnation of numbers of Protestant officials, one of whom, James Pike, the Episcopal Bishop of San Francisco and a long-time Planned Parenthood supporter, also demanded to know if the church's policy was binding on Catholic candidates for political office.

The question had special resonance, of course, because the first Catholic candidate since the defeat of Al Smith in 1928 was seeking the presidency. Sen. John F. Kennedy of Massachusetts immediately told James Reston of *The New York Times* in a telephone interview that it was absolutely not in America's interest to promote birth control overseas—that it would be a "mean paternalism…a great psychological mistake for us to appear to advocate limitation of the black or brown or yellow peoples whose population is increasing no faster than in the United States." But Kennedy was equally insistent, on this and subsequent occasions, as the issue dogged him through the campaign the following year, that he would act only on the basis of what he considered to be in the public interest, without regard to his private religious views or the public position of his church. Making birth control a condition of foreign aid was never the real issue. When later pressed about what he would do if foreign governments like India affirmatively requested American assistance, or if Congress took the initiative, he retreated somewhat from his initial formulation but insisted that the likelihood of any President ever having to sign a bill authorizing expenditures on birth controls as "very remote indeed" and repeated that, whatever he did, his actions would be based solely on his assessment of the national interest. Even Eleanor Roosevelt was willing to endorse this position.

Kennedy could afford to beg the more pointed question of cooperative assistance programs, because President Eisenhower, fearing the potential divisiveness of the matter on the upcoming campaign, then repudiated the Draper Commission recommendations, much to the surprise and dismay of its members. After the Kennedy story broke, the President responded with unusual bursequeness to a reporter's inquiry by saying he could not imagine a less "proper political or governmental activity or function or responsibility" than for the United States to promote family planning abroad. He advised instead that concerned foreign governments seek assistance from private groups.

From Tucson, Margaret announced immediately that she was prepared to debate Eisenhower in order to "straighten him out" on the question of family planning, and her statement made headlines as far away as Tokyo. She then wrote a letter to *The New York Times* insisting on the importance of population control to future world peace and protesting the position of the Catholic Church. Prominently displayed in the Sunday edition, it provoked an immediate exchange between Senator Kennedy and reporters on that morning's edition of "Meet the Press" in which he again protested his independence.

Shortly after the program aired, the telephone rang at Margaret's house, and her old friend, Norman Thomas, was on the line. Margaret almost always stayed clear of partisan politics and quietly cast her Presidential ballot for Thomas, but the lively, perennial candidate of the Socialist Party urged her to become more actively involved on this occasion by pointing out to the press that Kennedy's longtime acquiescence to church interference during successive referenda on the question of reforming punitive birth control laws in Massachusetts surely belied his claims of autonomy. She rose to the challenge and immediately wrote Kennedy a letter along the lines Thomas suggested, but when she never received any response, she seems to have dropped the matter. Nor did Thomas pursue it, his restrained, gentlemanly demeanor in campaign being legendary.

Had Margaret been twenty years younger, or perhaps just a bit healthier, she might have been less reticent. She did create international headlines once again after Kennedy's nomination, when she baldly announced that she would leave the country if he were elected, but the empty threat of an old woman in the middle of a hot summer hardly stirred up much of a fracas. Just two weeks before the November vote, however, three Catholic bishops in Puerto Rico issued a pastoral letter instructing their parishioners to oppose the island's popular incumbent governor, Munoz Marin, because he had endorsed public schools and birth control, and Washington's political reporters went crazy over the story. Catholic spokesmen in Washington quickly repudiated the statement, and Kennedy himself condemned the church-state interference, but according to the memoir by his aide, Theodore Sorensen, he knew he had been hurt. "If enough voters realize that Puerto Rico is American soil," Kennedy is reported to have said, "this election is lost."

It was, indeed, won with just over 100,000 votes out of more than 68 million cast, and various pollsters estimated that from 1 to 2 million voters deserted Kennedy in the last two weeks of the election when the Puerto Rican story broke. For the second time in her life, Margaret voted for a Republican Presidential candidate and announced publicly that religion was the reason. She then added that mutual friends were assuring her that the new President had an open mind and promised to give him a year before making good on her threat to find another place to live.

The election controversy generated a windfall of publicity for birth control advocates. More Americans than ever before became aware of the world population problem. *Reader's Digest,* with some 15 million subscribers, featured a flattering biographical portrait of Margaret. NBC News tried to match the ratings of the CBS show on India with an investigative piece of its own on Hong Kong. *Newsweek* prepared a special report on the "crisis," and Vance Packard wrote a best-seller on the subject. Planned Parenthood presented a statement of conviction about overpopulation to the Untied Nations, signed by 200 internationally prominent individuals, including thirtyeight Nobel laureates. Even the once publicity shy Population Council contracted with a public affairs agency and issued a pamphlet called *This Crowded World.*

According to population policy analyst Phyllis Tilson Piotrow, the election of a Catholic President, publicly committed to analyzing the matter in terms of objective national interest—rather than as a religious or moral dilemma—put great pressure on all parties to work toward reconciliation. Perhaps, as President Eisenhower is reported to have said privately, a Catholic in the White House might be able to accomplish what a Protestant could not.

For the time being, however, the matter remained in private hands. Incensed by Eisenhower's public disavowal of the Draper Panel, Hugh Moore called a group of prominent citizens together in Princeton, New Jersey, in March of 1960 to consider what could be done voluntarily to address the population issue. Margaret promised to be there—"if humanly possible, if I have to crawl," as she put it. Though quite nervous about her health, she did make the trip and brought along $25,000 from Martha Rockefeller toward the $100,000 that Moore put together to launch a World Population Emergency Campaign, which would run for two years and generate a membership of 10,000 individuals and more than a million dollars in funding for the International Planned Parenthood Federation.

So long as Moore could attract powerful men to the cause, like General Draper and Lammot duPont Copeland, of the industrial family, Margaret was willing to forgive the Dixie Cup king his rhetorical excesses, not to mention the fact that he was already on his fourth wife, whom she not so incidentally described as "beautiful and young," in a gossipy letter to Mrs. Rockefeller. Moore, in turn, recognized the mass marketing potential of Margaret's name, and asked her to sign a direct mail fund-raising appeal and a full-page advertisement in *The New York Times,* after agreeing to her demand that the population crisis be postured as a humanitarian concern, with all references to the threat to Communism excised from the text. Responses came back with small contributions and tender greetings from women who had followed Margaret's career throughout the years—one who first heard her speak in 1916 and then organized clinics in California, another who said that reading *Woman and the New Race* had changed her life. An ever vigilant Federal Bureau of Investigation also noticed the salutation and, seeing

Margaret's name, transmitted a copy of the letter to the agencies in its regular security network. Only one apparently bothered to respond. A baffled William Josephson, then the young and earnest general counsel at the Peace Corps, took the time to note that he didn't think the matter warranted any further investigation.

Had Margaret known about this internal communication, the interest J. Edgar Hoover and his agents demonstrated in her might have meant a great deal, or, at least, given her a good laugh. Alone much of the time in Tucson, she was drinking more and taking stronger doses of Demerol to ease her pain. In March of 1961, a fund-raising consultant hired by the World Population Emergency Campaign orchestrated a tribute in New York to honor her forty-fifth anniversary as a birth control advocate. The tragic deterioration in her physical and emotional condition is evident in the handwritten note she sent in response to his invitation, admitting that she was not "so rugged" as in the past but nevertheless hoped she could "pep up" and come to New York for the celebration. With the help of a secretary, she then wrote a more cogent reply admitting no less poignancy: "I cannot tell you how my heart goes out to you for all you are doing. As a matter of fact, you are the only one in recent years who has any knowledge of the history of the Movement or that Margaret Sanger had anything to do with it. It is to laugh, but that is the way it is."

The notable British scientist Sir Julian Huxley chaired the event, which included a dinner and a symposium of eminent scholars, physicians, and policymakers speaking about world population. Agnes Meyer, who had died in the interim, gave the initial gift that made it all possible, and Katherine McCormick provided the basis of a $100,00 endowment for IPPF to be maintained in Margaret's name. An eloquent testimonial was prepared, including greetings from friends in thirty-five countries and a charming printed program with old photographs of Margaret. *The New York Times* made her its "Woman in the News," while to everyone's surprise, an article in the Catholic journal, *America,* for the first time acknowledged the existence of an international population problem but rejected the position of those who would "Sangerize" the world, contending that so long as Communist countries were encouraging growth, so should nations in the free world.

Stuart Sanger accompanied his mother to New York, and he assisted her to the podium to deliver a brief message of thanks. Emotionally overwhelmed and exhausted by the experience, however, she then nodded off to sleep at the dais and was returned immediately to her hotel room. It was her last appearance in public.

Back in Tucson a new doctor slowly weaned Margaret of her addiction to painkillers and limited her to one drink a day. By the testimony of friends, she was serene and at peace with herself as she had not been in years, but even as she grew stronger and more coherent, she could no longer live alone or manage her own fairs. Barbara Sanger dutifully came in every day to check up on her, but the Sanger girls were grown and had left Tucson, and Stuart seemed utterly incapable of dealing with the dependency of the figure whose difficult but forceful presence had dominated his life for so long. Neither he nor Grant ever told their mother of William Sanger's death at the age of eighty-seven from a heart attack on July 25, 1961. And Bill, in turn, never saw the poignant letter Margaret had written forty-two years earlier to be given to him after her own death. She had looked at it herself on several occasions, but never made any practical arrangements to ensure its delivery.

Olive Byrne Richard had retired to Tucson and stopped by regularly to assist Margaret with correspondence and other domestic chores. She remembers her sitting for hours in the corner of the large living room she had furnished in a minimalist Oriental style. All of a sudden, Margaret began to fill every available surface with old photographs of family and friends that seemed strangely out of place in these spare surroundings. Yet they provided the only company she could find.

In the fall of 1961, Ellen Watumull asked friends and former colleagues to join her in a friendly conspiracy. Margaret was feeling much better than in the past, but there are times when she feels completely forgotten, Watumull confided. Would they write occasionally with news of what was happening in their part of the world? Would they bring some problem to Margaret's attention, ask her advice, needle her a bit about some controversy? Would they send her a book review, a news clipping, or just a post-card?

A typical response came from John D. Rockefeller III, who had just received the Lasker Award for family planning and had also spoken in Rome before a United Nations Assembly. "In these two public appearances I realized that what I was doing was following in your footsteps—in a small way helping to carry forward the tremendously important work for which you were so largely responsible," he wrote. And then, lest the letter sound too programmed, perhaps, he added a personal note. "I remember so well how much my mother and father used to enjoy their visits with you in Arizona. They spoke of you often. My personal regret is that our paths have not crossed more often."

Within two weeks, Rockefeller received two responses to his greetings. The first carried on obsequiously about the "splendid heritage" of the Rockefeller family. The second, asking for money to fund the deficit of the Margaret Sanger Research Bureau in New York, demonstrated that Margaret might be down but could not yet be counted out. Rockefeller instructed his staff to investigate why Planned Parenthood in New York was not taking responsibility for the clinic, which seemed to him only proper, but on the grounds that he did not support freestanding medical institutions, he never made a contribution and never wrote again.

In his remarks at the Sanger anniversary symposium, Marriner Eccles, a former New Dealer and chairman of the Federal Reserve, had predicted that the rate of world population growth might prove more explosive than the atomic or hydrogen bomb. The alarmist rhetoric occasioned an editorial in *The New York Times,* which called on the Kennedy administration to accept the recommendations of the Draper Report and assist friendly nations in population planning at their request. Key appointees at the State Department did not disagree with this proposal in principle but determined, after extensive internal debate, that active intervention by the United States was simply not "feasible" because of religious and social obstacles at home. A compromise strategy recommended that the federal government quietly support more extensive demographic and medical research through the National Institutes of Health, but a report proposing a preliminary agenda for work by the agency was then quashed in 1962 by politically timid advisers to the President. All this in spite of an increasing recognition that the Kennedy Administration's desire to leave a strong and innovative foreign aid program as its legacy was being compromised by the magnitude of a staggering world population problem. Further capitulation to fears of inciting the Catholic Church was also evident that year at the United Nations, where the United States at first supported, but then, by abstaining on a necessary second vote, helped to defeat, a resolution introduced by the government of Sweden permitting technical assistance in population planning to nations requesting it.

As the Kennedy administration waffled, however, an extraordinary mobilization of private resources for addressing the population issue took place. The budget of the Population Council expanded fivefold, while the Ford and Rockefeller Foundations got ready to make a major commitment of their own resources to programs in the population field. Following its dramatic successes in fund- aising and public relations, the World Population Emergency Campaign merged with the Planned Parenthood Federation of America on the grounds that a single organization marketing family planning at home and abroad would be more effective. Cass Canfield, the highly considered and well-connected head of the publishing firm of Harper and Row, who was already serving as chairman of Planned Parenthood's board, took charge of the combined organization. The venerable Alan Guttmacher of Mr. Sinai Hospital in New York then retired from medical practice and replaced William Vogt as a full-time president and chief executive officer.

Within a year, Planned Parenthood clinics in the United States would be serving nearly 200,000 patients, a gain of more than 30 percent. With the introduction of the pill, caseloads expanded so fast that some facilities had to impose limitations on service because of lack of funds. About 20 percent of this clientele was on public assistance, and the need for expanded distribution of services to indigent women through tax-supported hospitals and welfare agencies quickly became apparent. In many areas of the country, however, there were no public institutions in place providing the sustained preventive health care that medical contraception required, so Planned Parenthood had no choice but to expand its services to fill in the gaps, a situation that continues today. To this end, the politically skillful and diplomatic Guttmacher announced his determination to eliminate the movement's elitist reputation by broadening the base of its constituency to include better representation from organized labor, ethnic groups, and racial minorities.

Meanwhile, from a political standpoint, the publication in 1963 of John Rock's book, *The Time Has Come, A Catholic Doctor's Proposals to End the Battle Over Birth Control,* was also especially important. Though the church hierarchy did not accept Dr. rock's inventive defense of the pill as a natural contraceptive, a deliberate effort was made at conciliation in public comments on the book by Richard Cardinal Cushing of Boston, who also met privately with Alan Guttmacher. Even more important, in Rome, Pope Paul VI appointed a commission of clerical and lay Catholics to review the subject. Its ostensible aim was to reconcile Catholic theology with the most current scientific expertise in family planning. Three years later, American newspapers would report rumors that the commission was struggling with a recommendation to leave the matter of choosing a specific birth control technique to individual Catholic conscience. These stories could never be confirmed, however, and the Vatican made no official announcement until the publication in 1968 of the papal encyclical *Humanae Vitae,* which suddenly reconfirmed the immutability of natural law doctrine. Because the commission had never been able to reach a consensus, the Pope simply reiterated the doctrine that "every marriage act must remain open to the transmission of life." Only natural laws and rhythms of fecundity might constrain fertility. Man does "not have unlimited dominion over his body in general...or over his creative faculties." The statement also expressed concern that artificial birth control was making men especially vulnerable to "infidelity and the general lowering of morality" and to the use of women as a "mere instrument of selfish enjoyment."

From a theological standpoint nothing had changed, but as a practical matter, no significant efforts would be made to enforce this reiteration of Catholic orthodoxy about contraception on secular social policy in America or elsewhere in the world. The situation politically would revert to quiet acquiescence, just as in the nineteenth century, the church-state battleground shifting, instead, to the debate over legalizing abortion.

Undoubtedly aware of the internal debate going on within the church, President Kennedy, in his last statements on population, hinted at the potential for a change of his administration's policy when he finally acknowledged the seriousness of population growth and a willingness to have the United States make better "information" about it available to the world. In July of 1963, the Senate Foreign Relations Committee chairman, William Fulbright of Arkansas, insulated from Catholic intimidation by his largely Protestant constituency, seized the initiative from the executive branch and added an amendment to the foreign aid bill specifically authorizing programs in population research and technical assistance. Within months, Adlai Stevenson, who was serving as ambassador to the United Nations, went before a Planned Parenthood audience to talk about the issue, and Dwight David Eisenhower publicly disavowed the position he had taken as President that family planning was not the government's business. Together with his predecessor Harry Truman, he then accepted the honorary chairmanship of a Planned Parenthood fund-raising campaign.

On December 16, 1963, only weeks after the Kennedy assassination, Pres. Lyndon Johnson signed the historic Fulbright bill into law. It was less than four years following Kennedy's prediction that the possibility of a President's ever having to authorize funds for family planning was remote.

Just several weeks earlier, the journalist Lloyd Shearer of *Parade* magazine had interviewed Margaret in her room at the House by the Side of the Road, a convalescent home in Tucson, where she had been living for the past year. He found her bedridden, but still spirited and "irrepressibly pedagogic," as he put it. She talked mostly about the past:

> Fifty years ago I realized what was coming – the population explosion we hear so much about today, women having more and more babies until there's neither food nor room for them on earth. And I tried to do something about it. Now I have thousands of people all over the world aware of that problem and its only possible solutions – family limitation and planned parenthood. But 50 years ago, what opposition I had: the law, the police, the government, even my own father! He was the most broad-minded Irishman I ever knew – Michael Higgins was his name. But he kept saying, "Margaret! Get out of it. Get out of it. The kind of nursing you're doing, the kind of project you're involved in – that's no life for a girl."

By Shearer's account, Margaret was happy to observe the change in the tide of international opinion about population and deeply satisfied that the American government had finally authorized the funding of family planning assistance abroad. He praised her for "having fearlessly faced imprisonment, condemnation and ostracism" and concluded: "To many persons, both her name and her views are still objectionable. But in the eyes of many she has lived to become a respected prophet in her own time."

Stuart Sanger sat in on the interview with his mother. It was one of her better days. She had been confined to a wheelchair or to bed since her return from Christmas dinner the previous year. That had been an especially festive occasion, because young Margaret Sanger, who married her second cousin, Olive Byrne Richard's son, Dom Marston, had just given birth to her first child, a little girl. Born on November 5, 1962, the baby was named Margaret but called Peggy after the child who would have been her great-aunt.

The matriarch of the family spent most of the day quietly reposing in bed, but when her great granddaughter was brought to her, she suddenly became animated and kept repeating: "Peggy's come back. Peggy's come back." She then ran her hands over the infant's head to discern her personality from its shape and contour, as Michael Higgins's phrenology books had instructed her to do so long ago. Observing this compelling but strange behavior, Margaret Marston despaired that her grandmother was growing more and more disoriented and confused. She did not then understand that her new baby had been born nearly forty-seven years to the day of little Peggy Sanger's death. She did not then know that her grandmother had stood by her own daughter's deathbed all those many years earlier actually believing she saw the light of Peggy's tiny soul ascending to the heavens, nor that she had kept up imaginary conversations with the dead child for years, fully anticipating that one day they would be reunited.

This extraordinary reunion with little Peggy Marston and her family turned out to be Margaret's last journey outside the nursing home. As they were driving back that day, Margaret Marston also remembers that her grandmother became quite agitated and began to cry, protesting that she wanted to go back to her own bed in her own home. It was an especially difficult moment. Stuart stopped the car and after a silence that seemed interminable told his mother firmly that she simply could not go home again, because her bed there was no longer made. The elementary reasoning quieted her down, but Stuart was distraught for days thereafter. It was the only time his daughter ever remembers seeing him express any visible emotion.

For the remainder of her life, Margaret was most often too tried to read or talk and had only infrequent visitors. She was only coherent some of the time and was able to remember the distant past far more clearly than anything recent. Old colleagues from the birth control movement and several friends from Tucson were deeply distressed that she had been placed in an institution by her family, and bending to criticism of the particular facility, Stuart had her transferred to a different one nearby called the Valley House and Convalescent Center. He then retired and moved with his wife to Mexico. Occasionally someone would come by to see Margaret, bearing a plate of her favorite chicken sandwiches, a birthday cake, or some other treat, but she had little appetite and seemed almost to waste away. Unable to sit up on her own any longer, she nonetheless had the presence to request that a nurse bring her a paper cup and straw so she could drink the champagne that Grant and Edwina brought when they came out to visit for Christmas in 1964. Young Anne Sanger admired one of the paintings she had done that hung on the wall of her little room, and she gave it to her as a gift with this message: "H.G. Wells says I was the greatest woman who ever lived." Yet when all six of Margaret's New York grandchildren lined up against the wall of her room to she could see them together, she couldn't keep track of their names.

Several months later the Planned Parenthood Center of Tucson sponsored a testimonial dinner in Margaret's honour and hailed her as "the woman of the century." She was unable to be there, of course, but 1,000 guests attended, including the Duke and Duchess of Windsor, the former New Dealer and American ambassador to England. Lewis Douglas, who lived in Tucson, and the wife of the Arizona Senator and Republican Presidential candidate, Barry Goldwater. They heard Dr. John Rock praise Margaret's remarkable ability to combine "practical action with idealism," while Mrs. B.K. Nehru, wife of the Indian ambassador to the United States, declared that she had "single-handedly carried the torch of responsible motherhood" to the women of India and all over a crowded world. The celebration received extensive news and editorial coverage in local papers, where embittered organizers called attention to the fact that neither Planned Parenthood—World Population in America nor the International Planned Parenthood Federation had sent an official representative. Nonetheless, there was some good news. Margaret's old friend Grace Sternberg had been campaigning for years to have her awarded an honorary doctorate from the University of Arizona and finally succeeded over the protest of several Catholics on the board of trustees. Announcement was made of the degree to be granted at commencement ceremonies in May.

In conjunction with the dinner, Ambassador Douglas and other leading Democrats in Arizona, including the United States Secretary of the Interior, Stewart Udall, also attempted to have President Johnson award Margaret Sanger a Presidential Medal of Freedom. Since the honor was intended to be nonpartisan, they lined up Republican support for the nomination from the conservative Goldwaters and the more liberal New York Senator, Jacob Javits. The publisher of Tucson's newspaper and many othe prominent Arizonans wrote to the White House and to the members of the Distinguished Civilian Service Awards Board of the United States Civil Service Commission, which handled the awards process. Pointing out that Margaret was terribly old and ill, they argued that she deserved to be honored before she died for the freedom she had struggled for so long to win for the world's women and families.

As a political issue, family planning had been put on hold because of the Kennedy assassination, the initiation of the Johnson administration, and the contentious election campaign of 1964. The White House was embroiled in historic civil rights legislation, and in the dramatic escalation of American military involvement in Vietnam, yet federal agencies were quietly beginning to address the matter. On the international front, the Agency for International Development assigned Dr. Leona Baumgartner, a former New York City health commissioner with a long-standing interest in birth control, to meet with government personnel and outside policy experts in anticipation of putting together practical programs, and at the State Department population officers were being assigned through the Alliance for Progress initiative to desks in every major country in Latin America. Secretary of State Dean Rusk and McGeorge Bundy, then chief White House foreign policy adviser, had also met with population activists, following the election. They rejected a proposal for the creation of a special commission but did see that a pledge was incorporated into President Johnson's State of the Union Message in 1965 to "seek new ways to use our knowledge to help deal with the explosion in world population and the growing scarcity in world resources." Four more specific references to the international population problem were made by the President that year, representing what the activists understood to be a "calculated escalation" to test public opinion and encourage government officials to act.

Meanwhile, on the domestic front there was even more demonstrable progress. During 1965, a dozen pilot projects were jointly developed by the new Office of Economic Opportunity and various Planned Parenthood affiliates around the country to bring contraceptive services to married indigent women as part of the Johnson administration's emerging War on Poverty. Only one major condition for this initiative was set by OEO administrator Sargent Shriver, the brother-in-law of the late President: that there be absolutely no publicity.

For the time being at least, President Johnson also insisted on keeping a cautious distance in public from family planning activists. White House staff firmly rejected all requests for formal meetings. They did not want the administration's policies to provoke resistance from Catholics and, in fact, maintained informal procedures for keeping in touch with key church officials about what was going on. Johnson himself wrote to Lew Douglas, who was a longtime personal friend, saying that he was "not unaware of the innovations and trail blazing" of Margaret Sanger but was constrained by the recommendations of the panel he had appointed to review award nominations. He clearly intended to do nothing.

No record of the panel's liberations can be found, but subsequent correspondence with Johnson refers to "certain difficulties" that arose in connection with the 1965 Presidential Medal of Freedom, and given the President's acknowledged sensivity to thinking within the Catholic Church, it is not hard to contemplate what those difficulties might have been. It was one thing to inaugurate pilot family planning programs, quite another to honour the country's best-known antagonist of Catholics.

In fact, the Johnson administration would move ahead on family planning with circumspection. Following Margaret's death, the President did agree to accept an award from Planned Parenthood for his international achievements which was given in her name, but he did not show up in person for the presentation ceremony. He was increasingly preoccupied by Vietnam and by the violence spreading through the country's urban ghettos, where black militants were becoming increasingly vocal. Johnson would not dramatically expand family planning assistance abroad or at home until legislated to do so by Congress in 1967. At that time, the historic Title X Amendment to the Foreign

Assistance Act authorized $35 million for family planning assistance to foreign governments, United Nations agencies, and private nonprofit organizations (including the International Planned Parenthood Federation), while amendments to the Social Security Act designated that no less than 6 percent of funds for Maternal and Child Health Services be spent on domestic family planning programs. These were not Presidential initiatives, however, but rather the work of a bipartisan coalition in the Senate, including Democratic Senators Fulbright and Gruening, who chaired extensive hearings, along with Joseph S. Clark of Pennsylvania, Joseph D. Tydings of Maryland, Alan Cranston of California, and the maverick Republican, Robert Packwood of Oregon. In the House, critical leadership was provided by two liberal Democrats, Morris Udall of Arizona and James Scheuer of New York and by two Republicans, Robert Taft of Ohio, and a newcomer from Texas. His name was George H. Bush, and he would remain a staunch advocate of reproductive freedom for women until political considerations during the 1980 Presidential elections accounted for one of the most dramatic and cynical public policy reversals in modern American politics.

Margaret did not live long enough to witness these developments. Happily, she did die with the comfort of knowing that the United States Supreme Court had made its historic decision in *Griswold* v. *Connecticut.* Though increasingly senile and frail, she also appeared to understand when told that the government of Japan in 1965 had granted her one of its highest honors, the Third Order of the Sacred Crown. She never learned, however, of a letter of August 11, 1966, sent by Lady Bird Johnson at the urging of mutual friends, wishing her good health and happiness on behalf of the President, though this informal communication was as close to official recognition as she ever received from her own country.

She died of arteriosclerosis on September 6, 1966, just a few days short of her eighty-eighth birthday. *The New York Times* ran a front-page obituary, and Edwina Sanger, traveling with her younger children in Greece, learned of the death from a cover photograph and story in *The Times of London.* On the floor of the United States Senate, Ernest Gruening mourned the passing of "a great woman, a courageous and indomitable person who lived to see one of the remarkable revolutions of modern times—a revolution which her torch kindled—the breakthrough which enables us to discuss birth control and the population explosion and to seek acceptable solutions."

A private funeral service was held two days later at St. Phillips-in-the-Hills, the Episcopal Church Margaret had occasionally attended in Tucson. Grant flew out with his oldest son, Michael, and Stuart came up alone from Mexico, but aside from a few local friends, no one else could make it. The Rev. George Ferguson delivered a eulogy that did not ignore Margaret's achievements on behalf of humanity but remembered her more for the marvelous sense of fun she brought to Tucson during the many years they knew each other, with her lively interests, festive parties and essential joy in living.

On September 21, 1966, the autumnal equinox, the extended Sanger family, along with numerous colleagues from the birth control movement, gathered for a memorial service at St. George's Church on Stuyvesant Square in New York, where Noah Slee had long worshipped. Included among the famous and powerful was Mrs. Rose Halpern, then a spry little lady of eighty, who had been one of Margaret's first patients in Brownsville and a member of the welcoming party that greeted her when she left jail.

The city's heaviest rainfall in sixty-three years produced gale-force winds and tortuous traffic congestion that day, and many of the mourners arrived late for the service in the large and beautiful church. A choir of twenty members robed in scarlet flanked an altar adorned with the flowers Margaret had most loved. Morris Ernst eulogized her in a light vein, enumerating her courageous accomplishments but emphasizing her wit and charm, and Hobson Pittman offered an even more personal remembrance. The new rector at St. George's had never met Margaret, but her long-devoted secretary, Florence Rose, sent along copies of past tributes, so he had good material with which to work. The weather provided him his best line. It was, he said, "a stormy day to end a stormy life."

But the last word must be Margaret's own.

In one of their final conversations, Margaret Marston asked her grandmother what she wanted said after she died. And Margaret said she hoped she would be remembered for helping women, because women are the strength of the future. They take care of culture and tradition and preserve what is good.

That, she hoped, would be her remembrance.

18

Birth Control Method

This is a book about options. It is based on the premise that there is no single method of contraception that is right for every woman. There is also no single method that will continue to be right for any one woman throughout her reproductive years.

Today there are more kinds of birth control to choose from than ever before. There are options that weren't even available in this country just a few years ago—such as the female condom, Depo-Provera, and Norplant. In addition, ongoing research and technological advances have transformed many "old" contraceptives, such as the Pill and the IUD, making them excellent choices for more women that ever before. Even some "natural" approaches to preventing pregnancy have gotten quite sophisticated these days. These techniques do not expose women to hormones and chemicals, but they do require considerable commitment and a solid base of knowledge about fertility if they are to be used effectively.

Many women are unhappy with the contraceptive they now use. If you are one of them, chances are good that you will be able to find a method that will work better for you, once you have all the facts you need at your fingertips. Without the facts, you might choose a contraceptive because one particular aspect of it sounds appealing, or because your best friend uses it—but that method might be a poor choice for you for any number of other reasons. Conversely you might not even consider a particular method that could be an excellent choice for you, simply because your mother or a friend had a bad experience with it, or because you saw or read an unfavorable story about it in the news.

In some ways the sheer number of options available today can, in and of itself, make picking the right contraceptive harder. Condoms, spermicides, diaphragms and cervical caps, pills and shots and implants, IUDs, and sterilization. From this almost bewildering array, how can you zero in on the single method that is right for you, right now? How can you know when it's time to change your method—since, as we have said, no single contraceptive will be the right choice for a woman throughout her childbearing years. If you're forced to stop using a particular contraceptive—due to health problems, say or a change in lifestyle—how can you decide what to try next? How can you make a truly informed decision?

Consider the Methods You've Tried in the Past

One good place to start is to take a minute to think about all of the contraceptive you've ever used—why you chose the methods you did, what you liked and disliked about each of them, and what made you stop using one method and switch to another.

Think About What's Most Important to You

There are a number of factors to consider when you're choosing a method of birth control. They include the following:

- The method's *effectiveness*
- Its *cost*
- Your *personality* and *lifestyle*
- Your *stage in life*
- Your *fertility*
- Your *risk of sexually transmitted diseases* (STDs)
- Your *partner's attitude toward birth control*
- Your *health*

Effectiveness

Birth control methods vary tremendously in how well they prevent unintended pregnancies. For example, fewer than one woman in one hundred will get pregnant in a year of using either the ParaGard IUD or Depo-Provera injections; compared with about twelve condom users in one hundred and approximately eighteen women out of every one hundred who choose the diaphragm. How much risk are you comfortable with? Exactly how sure do you need to be, for your own peace of mind, that you won't get pregnant? Have you thought about what you would do if you did have an unplanned pregnancy? This isn't an easy issue to consider, but it should be a part of your contraceptive decision making.

The chart on the next page shows how often women become pregnant accidentally when they're using the various methods of birth control. You may be surprised, when you look at it, to see how certain methods rate. You may also be surprised by how big a difference there is between the most effective and the least effective methods.

Percentage of women experiencing a contraceptive failure during the first year of typical use and the first year of perfect use and the percentage continuing use at the end of the first year, United States

Method	*% of Women Experiencing an Accidental Pregnancy within the First Year of Use*		*% of Women Continuing Use at One Year*
	Typical Use	*Perfect Use*	
Chance	85	85	
Spermicides	21	6	43
Periodic Abstinence	20		67
Calendar		9	
Ovulation Method		3	
Sympto-Thermal		2	
Post-Ovulation		1	
Withdrawal	19	4	
Cap			
Parous Women	36	26	45
Nulliparous Women	18	9	58
Sponge			
Parous Women	36	20	45
Nulliparous Women	18	9	58
Diaphragm	18	6	58
Condom			
Female (Reality)	21	5	56
Male	12	3	63
Pill	3		72
Progestin Only		0.5	

Method	% of Women Experiencing an Accidental Pregnancy within the First Year of Use		% of Women Continuing Use at One Year
	Typical Use	Perfect Use	
Combined		0.1	
IUD			
Progesterone T	2.0	1.5	81
Copper T 380A	0.8	0.6	78
LNg 20	0.1	0.1	81
Depo-Provera	0.3	0.3	70
Norplant (6 Capsules)	0.09	0.09	85
Female Sterilization	0.4	0.4	100
Male Sterilization	0.15	0.10	100

Emergency Contraceptive pills: Treatment initiated within 72 hours after unprotected intercourse reduces the risk of pregnancy by at least 75%.
Lactational Amenorrhea Method: LAM is a highly effective, *temporary* method of contraception.
Source : (Hatcher R.A., Trusell, J, Stewart F, Stewart GK, Kowal D, Guest F, Cates W, Policar MS. Contraceptive Technology, New York: Irvington Publishers, Inc., 1994)

Another very important thing to notice about this chart is that it has two separate columns, one listing pregnancy rates for "typical use" and the other for "perfect use." For some methods—look at condoms, for example—there's a big difference between the numbers in those two columns. Typically, if one hundred couples used condoms for one year, twelve women would get pregnant. If, on the other hand, those one hundred couples used this method perfectly—*exactly according to instructions every time they had sex*—just three women in one hundred would be expected to get pregnant. For other methods, such as Norplant, the numbers in the two columns are exactly the same. Why? Because once the tiny hormone-filled tubes are implanted in a woman's upper arm, it is impossible to "forget" or misuse this method.

Cost

Here, too, the range is enormous. Norplant implants cost about $360, a diaphragm about $20 (not including a doctor's office visit in either case). Two methods that cost virtually the same when averaged out over time can hit your pocketbook very differently. For example, Norplant and tubal ligation (female sterilization) and vasectomy (male sterilization) are all quite expensive, and you have to pay for them up front. (Some of the cost may be covered by insurance). With methods like condoms and spermicides, on the other hand, you pay as you go, buy only as much as you need, and only when you need it. We have included a cost-comparison chart so that you can see some of the differences at a glance.

Cost of contraceptive methods, based on assumption of 100 acts of intercourse annually

Method	*Unit Cost($)*	*Annual Cost($)*	*Comments*
Cervical Cap	20 plus 50–150 for fitting	Cost of spermicide: 85	
Male Condom	0.50	50	Add cost of spermicide if used
Female Condom	2.50	2.50	Add cost of spermicide if used
Diaphragm	20 plus 50–150 for fitting	Cost of spermicide: 85	
Depo-Provera	35/injection	140	
IUD	120 plus 40-50 for insertion/lab tests	160 for Progestasert; 20 for Cu T 380A if retained 8 years*	
Norplant	350/kit plus 150–250 for insertion/removal	130–170 if retained 5 years*	5-year cost: 650–850
Pill	10–20/cycle	130–260	
Spermicides	0.85/application	85	
Sponge	4/pack of 3	133	

*Norplant and Cu T 380A have considerably higher annual costs if devices are removed prior to expiration; however, Wyeth Laboratories will refund cost of implants if removed before 6 months.
Soure : (Hatcher R.A., Trusell, J, Stewart F, Stewart GK, Kowal D, Guest F, Cates W, Policar MS. Contraceptive Technology, New York: Irvington Publishers, Inc., 1994)

Personality and Lifestyle

A lot of what you should consider when it comes to your lifestyle and personality is directly linked to the issue of "perfect use" versus "typical use", because some methods of birth control are a lot easier to use correctly than others.

Are you the type who can remember to take a birth control pill every single day? Would you really be willing and able to take your temperature every morning before you get out of bed, as one "natural" method requires? Do you have the discipline to put in your diaphragm or Reality condom every time you have sex? If you are fairly orderly, detail oriented, and motivated, you probably will remember to take your pills, and you might even enjoy the challenge of tracking your temperature as a means of natural fertility control. If, on the other hand, you are more spontaneous or the type who always loses her keys, you are probably less likely to do well with these methods.

Now consider the other end of the convenience spectrum: Would you be thrilled to simply go to the doctor for a shot of Depro- Provera every three months and basically forget about birth control in between? Or what about having Norplant's six tiny tubes of hormone implanted in your upper arm to prevent pregnancy for up to five years? If convenience is a top priority, you could even choose a ParaGard IUD, which, once inserted, works for up to ten years.

Some women don't like to take pills. If you're one of them, you're not going to do well on oral contraceptives, no matter how perfect a match this method might be otherwise. Similarly if you hate shots, Depo-Provera is not for you. Some women don't feel comfortable touching themselves, so the diaphragm or cervical cap would not be good choices for them. There is no right or wrong here. The only issue is how well a particular method suits *you.*

Consider your schedule and the demands of your school or work. If, for example, your job requires a lot of long-distance travel or changing shift hours, it may be hard for you to take birth control pills regularly. (They work best when taken as close to once-every-twenty-four-hours as possible). If you have a baby or small children, you know that irregular hours and unpredictable schedules come with the territory, so your birth control choice should be as simple and foolproof as possible. If you and your partner have sex mostly on weekends, maybe a cervical cap (which can be left in place for forty-eight hours) would be the perfect choice; while the daily hormone dose of Norplant or Depo-Provera, or even the Pill, might strike you as contraceptive overkill.

Stage in Life

Most women should expect to use several different types of constraception during their reproductive lifetimes. After all, this is quite a span of years when you think about it, stretching from your first period, at about age eleven, to your last, at about age fifty-two.

Typically women will probably go through three basic stages during their child-bearing years:

The early years of sexual activity. During, this stage, women are at peak fertility (so they need a highly effective method), but they're often not yet ready to have children (so they also tend to be concerned about finding a method that has a low risk of jeopardizing their ability to conceive in the future). They may also need to be wary of sexually transmitted diseases, including AIDS.

The childbearing years. At this stage you may need a contraceptive that is safe to use while you're nursing a baby, for example, or one that's readily reversible so that you can stop and start using it easily between planned pregnancies.

After kids. At this point in life you've had all the children you want, but you're still fertile and still sexually active.

You might now opt for a method that wouldn't have been a consideration earlier, such as tubal ligation, or vasectomy for your partner.

These days of course there are practically as many variations on this basic theme as there are individual women. The first stage might last until your late thirties, if you haven't found the right man or if you're putting off having kids to concentrate on your career. you might decide you never want to have children. On the other hand you might marry your high school sweetheart, have three kids in your twenties, and be done with childbearing by the time you're thirty. Or you might have gotten divorced, fallen in love again, and be eager to have more children. No matter what path you end up traveling in life, however, the point remains the same: What you will look for in a contraceptive is likely to be quite different when you're eighteen or twenty-three than it is when you're thirty-five, and different again when you're forty-five.

The chart on the following pages shows how popular various methods are among women at different ages. Condoms, for example, are used most frequently by younger women. Sterilization steadily gains users as women get older. The Pill is most popular with women in the middle of their childbearing years.

Fertility

There are a number of factors that determine how fertile you are; that is, how likely you are to get pregnant. Your age is just one of them. (In general, fertility is highest from about the late teens to the midthirties, declines slowly until age forty or so, then drops more quickly after that).

Other factors that indicate how likely you are to be fertile include the following:

- Sex more often than two or three times a week, which increases the odds that there will be live sperm in your reproductive tract when you ovulate (release a mature egg from your ovaries).
- Regular periods, which would tend to indicate that you are ovulating regularly.
- Intercourse with a man you know is fertile. In other words if he's fathered children before, he's probably physically capable of doing so again.
- Previous pregnancy. While this is no guarantee of continued fertility, it does show that you were able to get pregnant in the past.

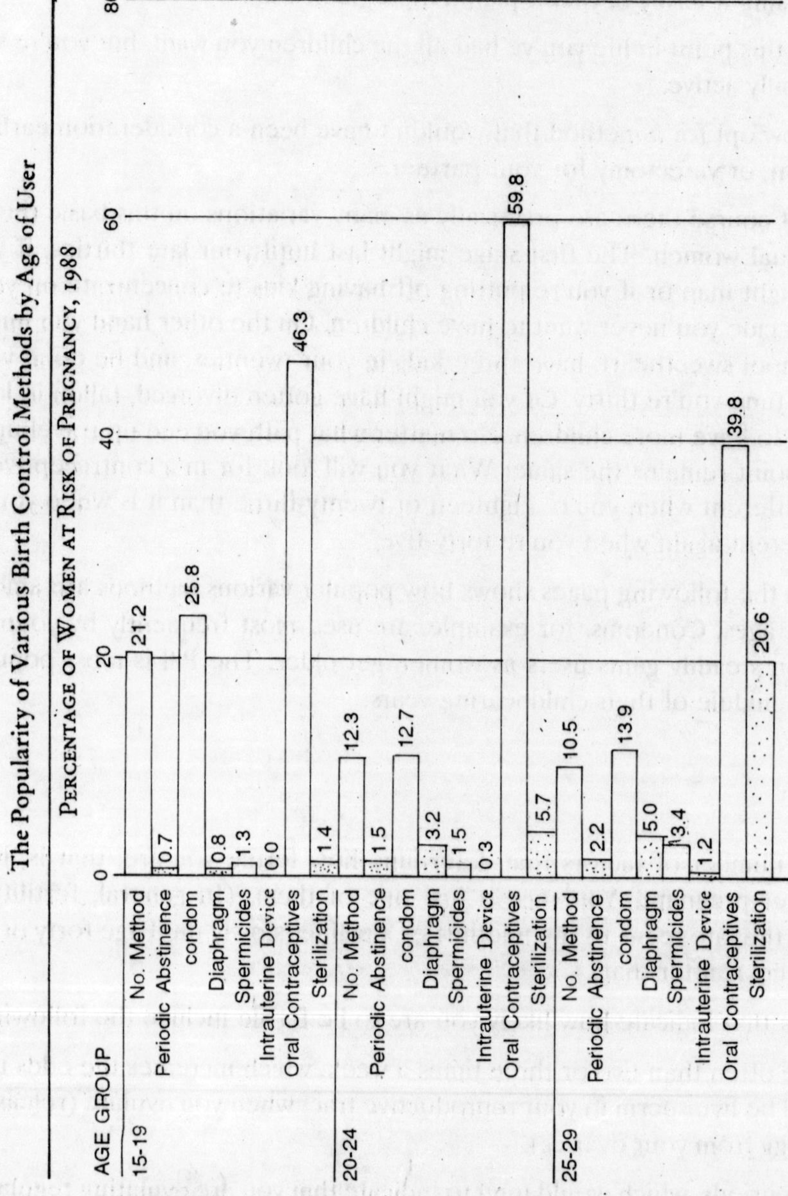

The Popularity of Various Birth Control Methods by Age of User

PERCENTAGE OF WOMEN AT RISK OF PREGNANCY, 1988

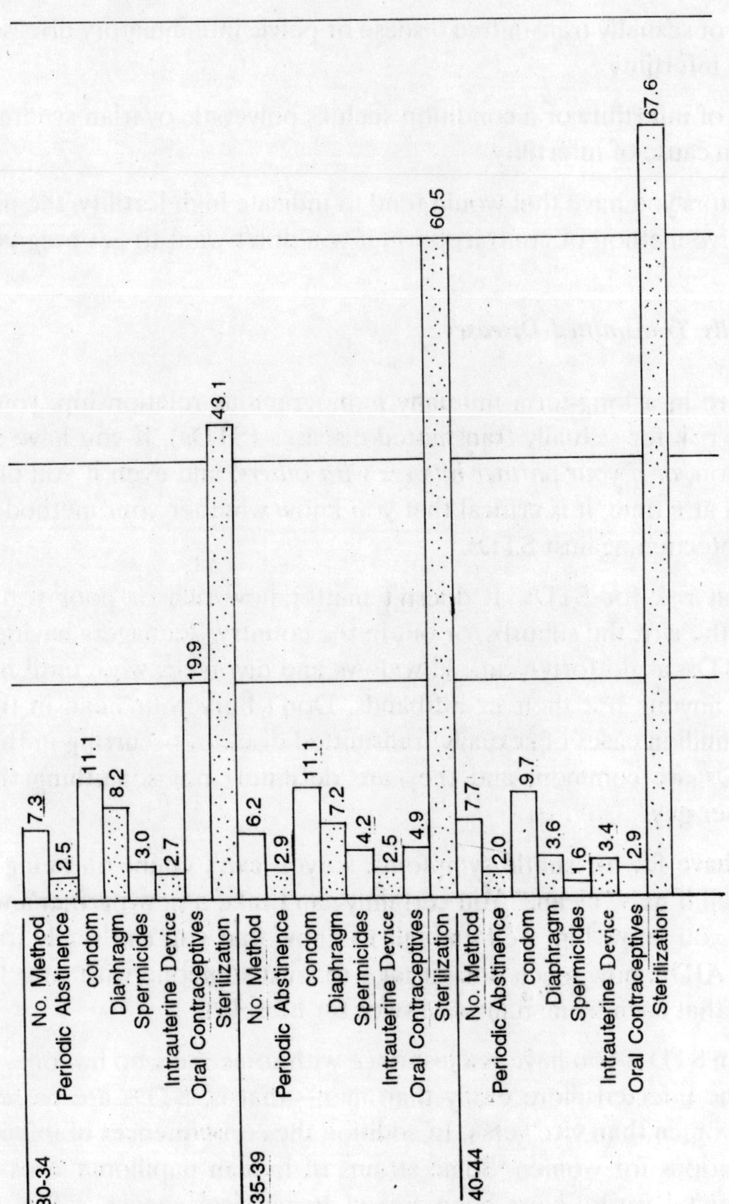

(Reproduced with permission of the Alan Guttmacher Institute from Susan Harlap, Kathryn Kost, and Jacqueline Darroch Forrest, Preventing Pregnancy, Protecting Health: A New Look at Birth Control Choices in the United States, *New York, 1991)*

Conversely some of the things that can indicate that you may be less likely to conceive include the following:

- Infrequent sex
- Skipped periods, irregular bleeding
- A history of sexually transmitted disease or pelvic inflammatory disease, which can cause infertility
- A history of infertility or a condition such as polycystic ovarian syndrome that is a known cause of infertility

The more factors you have that would tend to indicate high fertility, the more you need a highly effective method of contraception if you don't want to get pregnant.

Risk of Sexually Transmitted Diseases

Unless you are in a long-term mutually monogramous relationship, you should consider yourself at risk for sexually transmitted diseases (STDs). If you have sex with more than one person, *or if your partner has sex with others,* and even if you only have sex with one person at a time, it is critical that you know whether your method of birth control provides protection against STDs.

Everyone is at risk for STDs. It doesn't matter how rich or poor you are, or whether you live in the city, the suburbs, or out in the country. Teenagers having sex for the first time get STDs, as do forty-year-old widows and divorcees who, until now, had never had sex with anyone but their ex-husbands. Don't bury your head in the sand: With more than 12 million cases of sexually transmitted diseases occurring in this country every year, STDs are common, and they are definitely not something that only happens "to the other guy."

Many STDs have few or subtle symptoms, so you can't count on being able to look at a man and tell if he's "clean." You certainly can't take a new partner's word for it, at least not until you know him well enough to know that you can really trust him. (And in this age of AIDS, how much does it take to trust someone with your life? An impossible question that each woman must answer for herself.)

You can get an STD if you have sex just once with someone who has one. In most cases women become infected more easily than men—that is, STDs are passed more easily from men to women than vice versa. In addition the consequences of infection are often much more serious for women. Some strains of human papilloma virus (HPV), which can cause genital warts, have been linked to cervical cancer. STDs such as chlamydia and gonorrhea can cause pelvic inflammatory disease, which can permanently scar the fallopian tubes and result in infertility. Herpes is incurable; and it can, in some

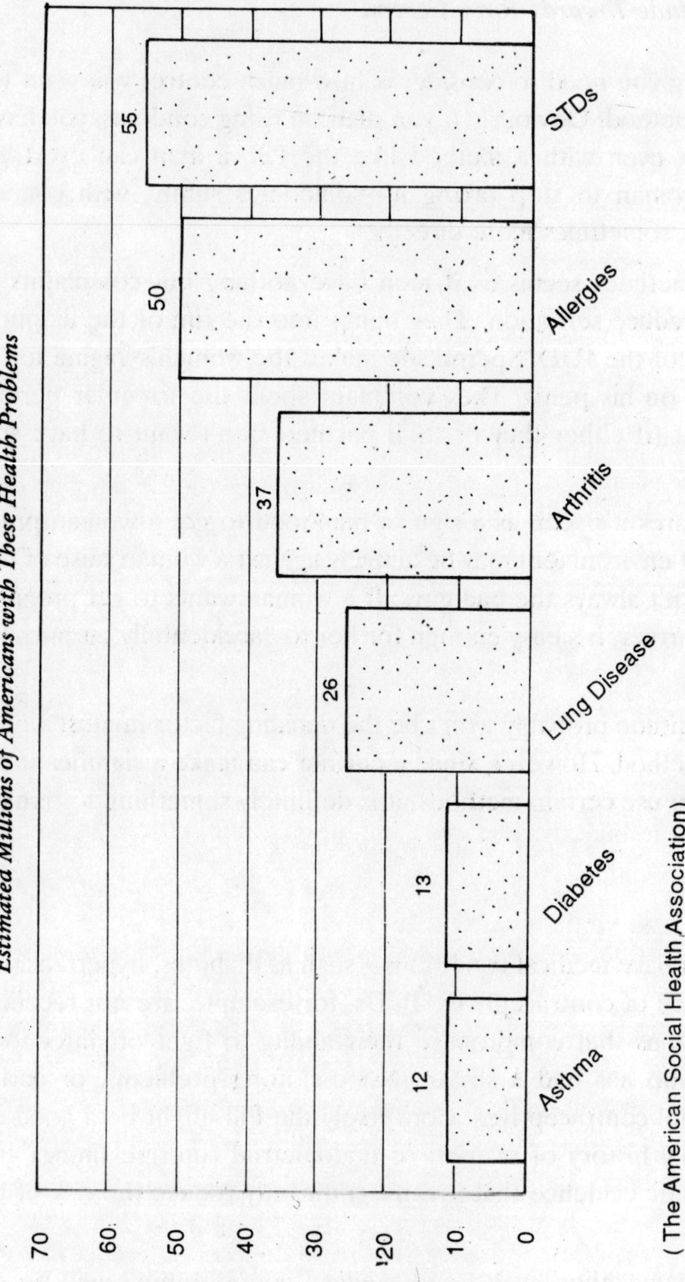
Sexually Transmitted Diseases: More Common Than Most People Think
Estimated Millions of Americans with These Health Problems
70
60
50
40
30
20
10
0
55
STDs
50
Allergies
37
Arthritis
26
Lung Disease
13
Diabetes
12
Asthma
(The American Social Health Association)

cases, cause serious infections in babies born to women with active outbreaks. And then there's AIDS, which as everyone knows by now, is both incurable and a killer.

Partner's Attitude Towards Birth Control

Another thing you need to consider is how much control you want to have over your birth control method. Obviously if you plan on using condoms, you have to have a willing partner. But even with a method like the Pill, a man can exert considerable influence over a woman to stop taking it—sometimes subtly, with comments about weight gain or acne, sometimes more directly.

In fact it sometimes seems as if men have nothing but complaints about birth control. Condoms reduce sensation. They bump into the rim of the diaphragm, or get poked by the string of the IUD. Spermicide makes the woman's vagina too slippery, or it irritates the skin on his penis. They complain about the irregular periods that can occur with Norplant (if either they or their partners don't want to have sex when the woman is bleeding).

In some cultures it's seen as a sign of manhood to get a woman pregnant. Men raised in this type of environment may be actively against a woman's use of birth control. (Of course men aren't always the bad guys: If a woman wants to get pregnant over the objections of her partner, it's easy enough for her to "accidentally on purpose" forget a pill or two).

The man's attitude probably won't be the deciding factor in most women's choice of a birth control method. However, since a partner can make a significant difference in how consistently you use certain methods, it is definitely something to think about.

Health

Many women have medical conditions—such as diabetes, hypertension, obesity—that limit their choice of contraceptives. IUDs, for example, are not recommended for women with conditions that compromise their ability to fight off infection, including AIDS. A woman who has had a stroke, blood-clotting problems, or certain cancers should not be on oral contraceptives. Conversely the Pill might be a good choice for a woman with a family history of ovarian or endometrial (uterine lining) cancer, since there is good scientific evidence that it can significantly reduce the risk of these malignancies.

These and many other health and medical considerations will be discussed in greater detail, as they apply, in the chapters on individual contraceptives.

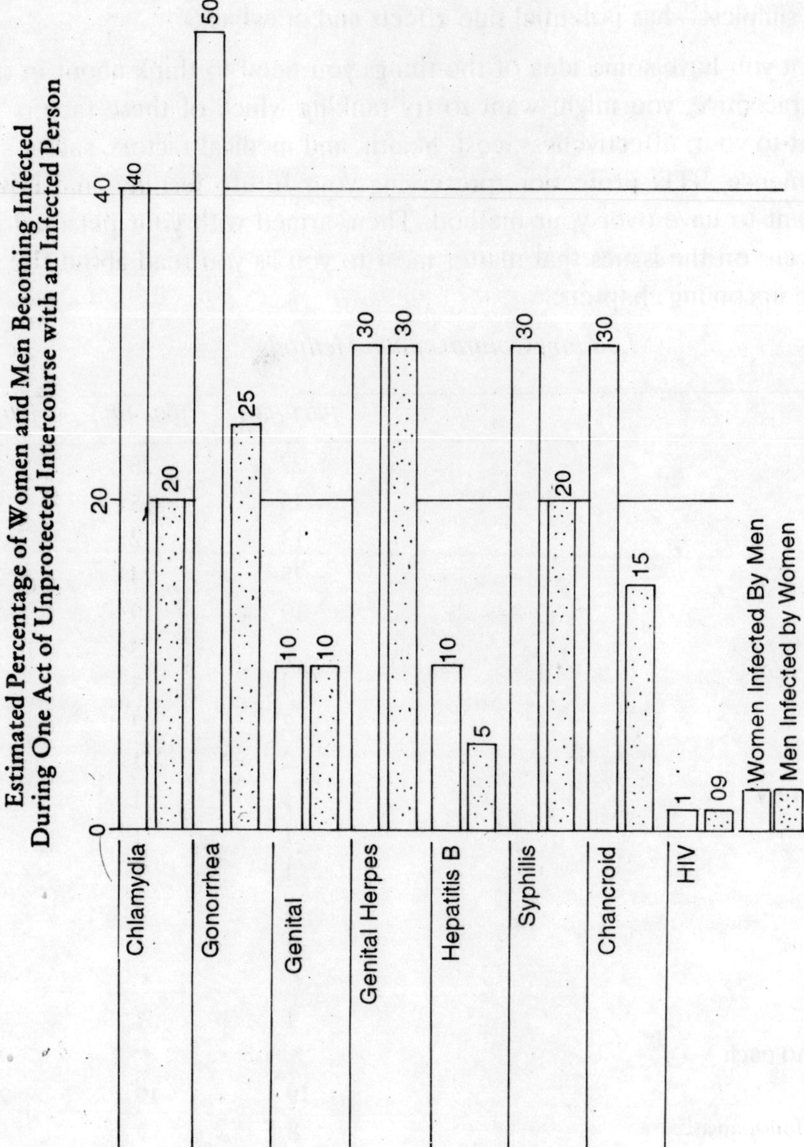

(Reproduced with permission of The Alan Guttmacher Institute from Susan Harlap, Kathryn Kost, and Jacqueline Darroch Forrest, Preventing Pregnancy, Protecting Health: A New Look at Birth Control Choices in the United States, *New York 1991)*

Zeroing in on the best contraceptive choice is often a matter of balancing the pros against the cons of several contenders, because just as there is no contraceptive method that's right for every woman, there is also no perfect contraceptive. Every method—even the most highly effective—has some failures. And every method—even the safest and simplest—has potential side effects and drawbacks.

Now that you have some idea of the things you need to think about in order to choose a contraceptive, you might want to try ranking which of these factors are the *most* important to your: effectiveness, cost, health, and medical factors, safety and side effects, convenience, STD protection, preserving your future fertility, and how much control you want to have over your method. Then, armed with your personal priority list, you can focus on the issues that matter most to you as you read about the various methods in the upcoming chapters.

Leading Contraceptive Methods

	1993 (%)	*1994 (%)*	*1995 (%)*
Sterilization	27	26	24
Tubal Ligation	15	15	15
Vasectomy	13	12	10
Pill	25	24	26
Condom	19	19	19
Withdrawal	6	5	6
Rhythm	3	3	3
Diaphragm	2	2	2
Sponge	2	1	1
Vaginal Suppository	2	1	1
Douche	1	1	1
Foam	1	1	1
IUD	1	1	1
Cream/Jelly alone	1	1	1
Cervical cap	*	*	*
Implant	1	1	1
Female Condom/Pouch	*	*	*
No method	19	19	20
Hysterectomy/Menopause	8	9	6
Pregnant	2	2	3
Trying to conceive	2	2	2

Finally, we've included one more chart. It shows you how popular various methods are today in the United States, and compares their use now to that in years past.

19

Body Basics

To really understand how birth control methods work, and to be able to use them correctly, you have to know a bit about the female body—both its anatomy (where things are and what they're called) and its physiology (how things work).

Female Body Parts—What's Visible on the Outside

The entire external genital area is often referred to in medical terms as the *vulva,* a Latin word that means "covering."

In sexually mature women this area is almost completely covered by the pubic hair. The bony rise just above the genitals, where the pelvic bones come together, is called the *mons pubis.* The outer folds of hair-covered skin, which protect and cover the vaginal area, are called the *labia majora,* which means "large lips" in Latin. Inside the folds of the labia majora are smaller, highly sensitive folds of pinkish skin known as the *labia minora,* or "small lips." At the top of the labia minora, an inch or so in front of the opening to the vagina, is the extremely sensitive, small knob of flesh called the *clitoris,* which plays a central role in sexual pleasure for most, but not all, women. The ring of tissue around the vaginal opening is the *hymen.* The hymen varies a great deal from woman to woman—it can be relatively thick and tough, or quite thin and easily stretched, or even virtually invisible. Because of these normal variations a sexual partner

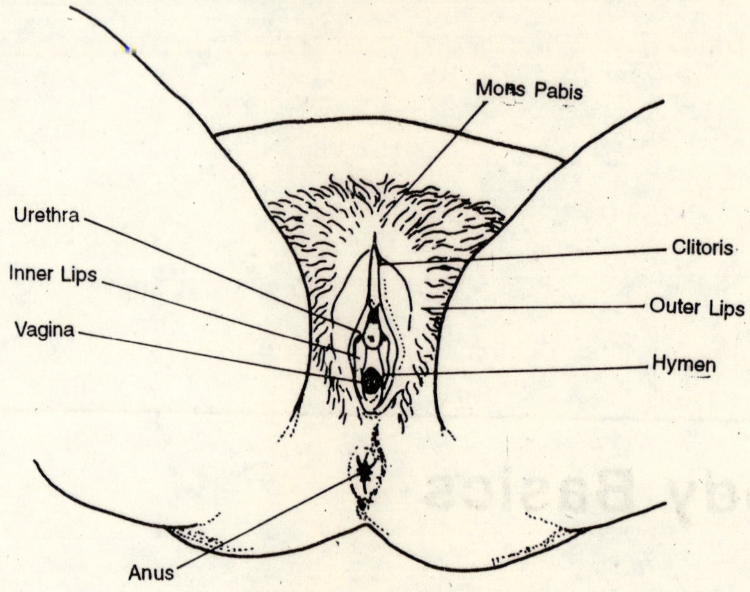

External Genital Area

can't tell whether a woman is a virgin by looking at her vaginal opening or by having sex with her. Even a doctor may not be able to tell during an examination.

The *anus,* which is the opening at the end of the intestinal tract, lies behind the vaginal opening. The opening of the *urethra,* the tube that carries urine from the bladder to the outside of the body, is between the vagina and the clitoris. This small slit is nearly invisible unless you gently pull its edges apart.

Inside the Female Body

In conspicuous contrast to the male reproductive system, most of the female organs of reproduction are on the inside of the body.

The *vagina* is the link between the external and internal organs of reproduction. In mature women the vagina is about four inches long and consists of soft, stretchy tissue that normally lies flat like a deflated balloon when there's nothing in it. During sexual excitement the walls of the vagina secrete lubricating fluid that allows the penis to slide into it more easily.

At the top, or internal end, of the vagina is the *cervix,* the narrow lower end of the *uterus* that juts out about an inch into the top of the vagina. You should be able to touch your cervix if you put a finger or fingers into the vagina and reach inward—it may feel

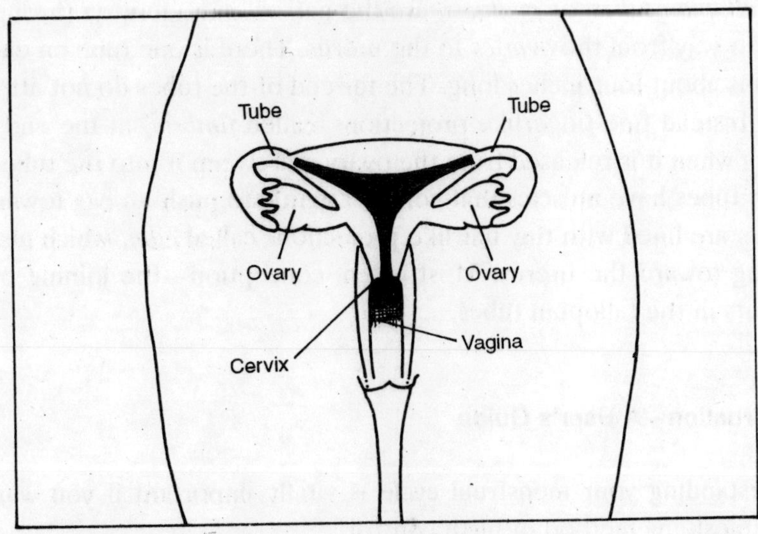

Interior Reproductive Organs

like a rounded bulge, harder than the surrounding vaginal tissue, with a dimple in its center. (Some people say the cervix feels a bit like the end of your nose.) Women who use barrier methods of birth control, such as the diaphragm and cervical cap, need to be comfortable locating the cervix inorder to check that these devices are in proper position.

The "dimple" in the cervix is the opening, or *os,* of the narrow canal that runs through the cervix from end to end. This canal opens and closes very slightly at different times of the menstrual cycle, and stretches wide during the delivery of a baby. Glands in the cervix produce most of the secretions that you may notice coming out of the vagina during the month. These secretions change with the ebb and flow of the menstrual hormones and can be used to help predict when a woman is fertile. It is the cervix from which your doctor collects cells when he or she takes a Pap smear.

The entire *uterus,* or womb, is approximately pear-sized and pear-shaped, with thick muscular walls that have the ability to expand enormously when a baby is growing within it. In your body the pear is upside down, with the narrow end being the cervix. The inside of the nonpregnant uterus is triangle-shaped. Each of the top two angles of the triangle leads to one of the *fallopian tubes* (or *oviducts*); and the bottom point of the triangle is the cervical canal. The tissue that forms the inner lining of the uterus is known as the *endometrium.* The endometrium responds to the stimulation of hormones during the menstrual cycle, first growing thicker and full of glands and blood vessels, and then, if conception does not occur, sloughing off and flowing down through the cervix and vagina in menstruation.

The *fallopian tubes,* or *oviducts,* are the narrow passage-ways through which eggs travel on their way from the *ovaries* to the uterus. There is one tube on each side of the uterus; each is about four inches long. The far end of the tubes do not attach directly to the ovaries. Instead fine fingerlike projections, called *fimbria,* at the end of each tube catch the egg when it is released from the ovary and sweep it into the tube. The walls of the fallopian tubes have muscles that contract gently to push an egg toward the uterus; and the tubes are lined with tiny hairlike projections called *cilia,* which also help sweep the egg along toward the uterus. Most often, conception—the joining of an egg and sperm—occurs in the fallopian tubes.

Menstruation – A User's Guide

Understanding your menstrual cycle is vitally important if you want to get the most from almost any method of birth control.

To give the most obvious example, knowing which days of the month you are most likely to conceive is critical to the successful use of natural methods of fertility control. Even users of barrier methods can significantly increase the odds that their method will protect them if they "double up"—using, for example, condoms plus a vaginal spermicide—during the most fertile part of each month.

It is also important for women using hormone-based contraceptives (such as Norplant or birth control pills) to know enough about the normal menstrual cycle so that they understand how and why their cycles are likely to change when they use these methods. For example amenorrhea (no bleeding) can be a normal side effect of Depo-Provera shots and Norplant. But if a woman isn't expecting and "misses" a period, she might well worry that her method has failed and she is pregnant. Another example: If a woman on oral contraceptives misses a pill or two, where she is in her cycle makes a big difference in how likely it is that her slipup will result in an unplanned pregnancy.

The Cycle Explained

Most women think about their menstrual cycles only in terms of bleeding—when their periods start and stop, how heavy or light, painful or cramp-free they are. This is natural, since bleeding is the only part of the cycle that is visible and tangible. But menstrual bleeding is actually the end result of a month-long chain of events that occurs inside a woman's body.

The whole point of the menstrual cycle—from an evolutionary perspective at least—is to prepare your body for a possible pregnancy. The preparation process itself is an extremely complex sequence that starts in the brain and culminates each month in either (a) pregnancy or (b) menstruation.

There are actually two main events, separate but inter-related, that occur during each menstrual cycle. One is that an egg ripens, or matures, and is released from the ovaries; the other is that the uterine lining thickens and prepares itself to support a pregnancy should that egg become fertilized. If the egg is not fertilized, the uterine lining is shed during menstruation, and the entire sequence of events begins anew.

The first day of bleeding (the visible evidence of the *end* of one menstrual month) is, then, also "day 1" of the *next* month's cycle. At that time *GnRH,* or *gonadotropin-releasing hormone,* a chemical messenger from the hypothalamus (an area of the brain just above the pituitary gland), sends a message to the pituitary to secrete FSH, or *follicle-stimulating hormone.* FSH prompts the ovaries to start ripening a number of eggs; and it stimulates the cells surrounding those eggs, called *granulosa cells,* to start to secrete *estrogen.* The estrogen from the granulosa cells stimulates the growth of the lining of the uterus (the endometrium).

By about day 6 of the menstrual cycle, as the follicles continue to develop, one somehow becomes the dominant follicle, the one that will release its mature egg at ovulation. (No one knows how the dominant follicle is "chosen" from the group of eggs that start to ripen at the same time.) As the follicles grow, and more and more estrogen is produced, the rising estrogen levels feed back to the brain, signaling the pituitary to produce less and less FSH.

About midcycle (day 14), the estrogen level peaks, triggering the secretion of *LH,* or *luteinizing hormone,* from the pituitary. LH has several different effects.

First, it causes ovulation, the release of the mature egg from the dominant follicle. After ovulation the egg travels down the fallopian tube to the uterus. If it is not fertilized by a man's sperm within approximately twenty-four hours, the egg will simply dissolve and its components will be reabsorbed by the body. Similarly the other eggs that had started to develop in their follicles will also simply wither away. If that seems like a waste of perfectly good eggs, consider this: A woman is born with about a million eggs in her ovaries. By the time she reaches puberty, about 300,000 viable eggs remain. Since she will need only about 400 to 500 to be released during ovulation in her lifetime, she has plenty of eggs to spare.

Second, LH also causes some of the granulosa cells around the follicles to start producing *progesterone* as well as estrogen. Once the egg has been released, the area where ovulation occurred becomes the *corpus luteum,* and continues to secrete estrogen and progesterone. Progesterone causes the lining of the uterus, now thick from the estrogen stimulation during the first half of the cycle, to change in preparation for the possible implantation of a fertilized egg. The uterine lining, or endometrium, becomes more fluid-filled, and has a higher sugar content for the nourishment of an embryo.

As the cycle continues, more and more progesterone is secreted by the corpus luteum, reaching a peak and plateauing off about eight to ten days after ovulation. Progesterone sends a feedback message to the brain, prompting the pituitary to secrete less LH. If no fertilized egg implants in the uterine lining, progesterone levels fall quickly. Without hormone support the built-up uterine lining sloughs off and menstruation begins.

If, on the other hand, the egg is fertilized and does successfully implant on the uterine wall, the developing *placenta* will take over the job of hormone production from the waning corpus luteum. In that case there will be no decline in hormone levels for the nine months of pregnancy. As long as the hormones remain high, the uterine lining does not shed and no new eggs will start ripening in the ovaries. After the baby is born, hormone levels drop, which is the signal that jump-starts the menstrual cycle into action once again.

Ectopic Pregnancy

An ectopic pregnancy occurs when a fertilized egg implants and starts to grow outside of the uterine cavity. Usually this occurs in one of the fallopian tubes. Very rarely a pregnancy will take hold in the abdomen, outside the uterus.

Ectopics occur, on average, in about one in two hundred pregnancies. They are more common in women who have had a previous ectopic and in those whose tubes have been damaged by infections or, sometimes, endometriosis. To the extent that birth control prevents fertilization, it also reduces the risk of ectopics, compared with women who are not using contraception.

Ectopics can be life-threatening if they are not caught in time. A growing pregnancy can rupture a tube and cause severe internal bleeding. It is important for all sexually active women to know the signs of ectopic pregnancy (a missed period followed by slowly worsening or sudden and severe lower abdominal pain, possibly accompanied by fainting) and seek medical attention promptly. It can sometimes be hard even for doctors to determine the cause of abdominal pain (distinguishing it from appendicitis, for example), but in women of childbearing age ectopic pregnancy should always be a prime suspect. One vital clue: a positive pregnancy test.

If an ectopic is diagnosed very early, it can be treated either surgically or chemically, with a drug called methotrexate. Often, in these cases, the tube can be preserved. Sometimes, especially if there is a delay in the diagnosis, the tube may be so damaged that it must be removed along with the ectopic pregnancy. A woman can go on to have a normal pregnancy after an ectopic, whether she has one tube left or two, although her risk of having another tubal pregnancy is increased.

What About Breastfeeding as Birth Control? Does It Work?

Yes, but...Nursing a baby causes the body to produce a hormone called prolactin, which does tend to suppress ovulation. However, only persistent, frequent breastfeeding keeps prolactin levels high enough to prevent egg development—a situation that is most common in cultures where women carry their babies with them during the day and let them suckle at will. In countries such as our own, where nursing mothers are often separated from their infants for hours at a time, breastfeeding as birth control tends to be less reliable. As soon as you start to feed your baby bottles of formula or solid food in addition to breast milk, you will probably start to ovulate again pretty quickly.

Also, if you think about it, you'll realize there's one rather major problem with relying on breastfeeding as birth control: Menstruation is the first visible sign that you're fertile again; but menstruation doesn't occur until *two weeks after you ovulate.* That means that by the time you might have gotten your first period after having had a baby, you could already be pregnant again.

When During the Menstrual Cycle Is Unprotected Sex "Safe"?

The sequence of events described above means that a typical woman can conceive from the day an egg is released (which happens about two weeks after the first day of your last period) until a day or so later, when that egg dissolves and can no longer be fertilized.

But you also must take into account the fact that sperm can live in a woman's reproductive tract for several days. Three days is perhaps typical, but studies have shown sperm survival for as long as a week. That means unprotected sex in the days *before* ovulation can also result in a pregnancy.

And add to that the fact that very few women have absolutely regular, "classic" twenty-eight-day cycles, and you start to see why it can be hard to figure out when it might truly be "safe" to have sex without birth control. (The ways in which natural methods of birth control attempt to predict "safe" times will be discussed in detail. Suffice it to say here that unpredictable variations in menstrual cycles and sperm survival are one reason this approach to birth control tends to have high failure rates. In order to work, natural methods need consistent use by couples who are committed to making them work.)

Menstrual cycles also don't stay the same over a woman's reproductive lifetime. For the first few months after menarche (the onset of menstruation, which occurs typically at about age eleven or twelve) periods tend to be irregular and unpredictable. The middle years of fertility (from about age eighteen to thirty- five) tend to have the most regular menstrual cycles, although even then they can be thrown off by such common occurrences as stress, illness, or significant weight gain or loss. Later in the reproductive years, after about age thirty-five or so, a slow decline in fertility can again cause menstrual-cycle shifts. At first these are likely to be as subtle as a slight shortening of the cycle, by perhaps a day or two. Later, after age forty, women tend to get more irregular and start skipping periods occasionally and unpredictably.

20

Talking to Your Doctor About Birth Control

Think of your doctor as a partner in your quest for the best possible method of birth control.

For the best results, the more you give—informationwise—the more you'll get. Your health care provider (he or she could be a private or HMO ob/gyn, a family practitioner, a college health service physician, or a counselor at a family planning clinic) may know a lot about human reproduction and contraception *in general*, but he or she doesn't know a thing about *you* as an individual.

So the more background information you can give your doctor, and the more open and honest you can be, the more likely it is that you will end up with a method that suits your lifestyle and your personality, as well as your physical needs.

Also the more you know about birth control before you walk into your doctor's office, the more you can learn from him or her. These days almost no health professional has the time he or she might wish to spend educating women about every aspect of each method.

If you come prepared, more time can be spent on your specific questions and concerns, and less on covering the basics.

Making It Easier to Talk

The things you need to discuss with your doctor are very personal, and therefore can be a bit awkward to talk about. To make opening up a bit easier, keep the following points in mind:

- No matter how complicated or unusual your circumstances, you're not likely to shock or surprise your doctor. He or she has almost certainly heard anything you have to say—and probably a lot worse—before. Remind yourself that your doctor is there to help, not to judge.
- Don't worry about terminology. You don't have to speak in technical or medical terms for your doctor to understand your concerns. Just use whatever words are comfortable, and be as clear and complete as possible.
- Anything that's important to *you* should be taken seriously by your health care provider. If you're concerned about the possibility of weight gain or acne if you go on the Pill, say so. If your boyfriend absolutely despises condoms, don't agree to use them when you know you know you really won't. If your current doctor recommends a diaphragm, and a past doctor told you you couldn't use one because of your tipped uterus, speak up and where the discrepancy comes from.
- Don't hesitate to ask for an explanation of any technical terms that aren't absolutely clear to you. Your doctor is not going to think you're stupid; he or she knows you don't have a medical degree. Medical lingo is so familiar to health workers that half the time they probably don't even realize they're speaking what sounds like a foreign language to the rest of us.
- And a final, very important point: Everything you tell your doctor—everything that goes in your medical records—is confidential. You don't have to worry about revealing such facts as, for example, a past abortion or about with a sexually transmitted disease that you've never even told your parents or your boyfriend or your husband about.

What Your Doctor Needs to Know About You

Many facets of your health history, both current and past, enter into the birth control decision. The following are some of the things your doctor will want to know about you to help you zero in on the best possible contraceptive method. As you read about them, you might want to jot down things that come to mind about your own health and medical history. Also write down any questions you may have for your doctor. That way you can take your notes with you to your appointment and have the information at your fingertips. By being prepared ahead of time, you can relax and concentrate on talking with your doctor instead of listening with half your attention while the other half is struggling not to forget when your last period started.

- *Menstrual cycle.* The date of your last period is just one of many things your health care provider will need to know about your menstrual cycle in order to help you choose an appropriate contraceptive. If your cycles are erratic and irregular, for example, fertility awareness methods may be almost impossible to use successfully. If your periods include heavy bleeding and severe cramping, the IUD is probably not a good choice because it can make those symptoms worse. The Pill, on the other hand, often brings about a lighter flow, fewer days of bleeding, and less cramping.

- *Fertility.* Have you ever been pregnant? If you have, were you trying to get pregnant, or trying not to (i.e., were you using birth control at the time)? If you got pregnant because of a birth control failure, do you know what went wrong, or were you using the method perfectly, as far as you know?

How important is it that you not get pregnant at this point in your life? Would an accidental pregnancy derail your college plans? Are you married and planning on having a family, just not quite yet? Are you very sure the three kids you have are enough, or would another sort-of-unplanned pregnancy not really be a big deal? Are you thirty-five and not yet married and extremely concerned about preserving your fertility for as long as possible? Each of these situations has very different implications when it comes to your birth control choice. And if your doctor understands where you're coming from, you are much more likely to end up with a contraceptive that will work well at this stage of your life—whatever that stage may be.

Age is a very important factor when it comes to choosing a birth control method, and it's one that probably isn't considered as much as it should be. For young, highly fertile women there is less margin for error in a birth control method. If you misuse or don't use contraception at this point in your life, or if you use a method that has a high failure rate even if it is used correctly, you may be quite likely to get pregnant. Older women, on the other hand, may be able to successfully "get away with" a contraceptive that's a bit less effective, such as a diaphragm or cervical cap, because they are somewhat less fertile.

- *Past birth control use.* Your doctor is going to want to know what methods you have used in the past, and why you stopped using them. Did you go off the Pill because you had breakthrough bleeding? If so, there's a good chance that a different formulation might not have the same side effects. Or did you stop because you broke up with your longtime boyfriend and didn't want to take medication every day when you knew you weren't going to be having sex with anyone for a while? Is there a particular method that interests you now that you want to ask the doctor about?

- *Your current sex life*. Are you married, single, divorced? Just now preparing for your first sexual relationship? Are you in a long-standing one-man-only relationship, or are you at a point in your life where you might have more than one partner? (This last includes "serial monogamy"—where a woman has sex only with her boyfriend, but over time has a number of sequential relationships).

These questions are important because of the risk of sexually transmitted diseases. Some birth control methods (particularly condoms, both male and female) offer very good protection from most STDs, including HIV, the virus that causes AIDS. Diaphragms and cervical caps provide less protection, the IUD none whatsoever. Hormonal methods, such as the Pill, Norplant, and Depo-Provera, don't keep women from catching infections, but because they make the cervical mucus thick and less penetrable, they may reduce the risk that germs will travel up through the cervix and possibly cause a tubal or pelvic infection. To protect themselves from infections, many women these days use condoms with new partners in addition to the pills they take for protection against accidental pregnancy.

Your current situation is also relevant in terms of the availability of your method. To work, your method has to be where you are when you need it. One of the major reasons for intended pregnancies among birth control users is that their method either wasn't available or wasn't used when they had sex. Take, for example, a college student who sometimes has sex with her boyfriend in her dorm room and other times sleeps over at his apartment. A stash of condoms and spermicide in both places might be an excellent option (and one that protects against both pregnancy and STDs when used every time you have sex). Birth control pills or a diaphragm are trickier. These methods will only work if she trains herself to carry them in the backpack that goes everywhere with her, instead of leaving them at home in her bedside table or bathroom cabinet.

- *Health conditions*. It is very important that your doctor know about any medical conditions you have or medications you take, since these can affect your choice of a birth control method.

Medical conditions are probably most relevant when it comes to hormonal methods, such as the Pill, Depo-Provera, and Norplant. For example, if you have a history of thrombophlebitis (blood clots and/or inflammation in the veins), breast cancer, or some types of liver diseases, these methods will probably not be an option. If you have uncontrolled high blood pressure or elevated cholesterol, the Pill may not be your best choice. Dilantin, taken to control epilepsy, can interact with oral contraceptives to make them less effective. On the other hand if you have endometriosis, it might actually get better if you take oral contraceptives. And if you are a young woman with a strong family history of ovarian cancer, a doctor might encourage Pill use, since it has been shown to significantly reduce the risk of this deadly disease.

There are also medical conditions that can affect your choice of nonhormonal contraceptives. If you take steroids, an IUD is not a good choice. This method would also most likely not be an option for women who have had PID (pelvic inflammatory disease, a serious infection that can cause infertility).

Are you bothered by recurrent cystitis? In some women diaphragms can make this problem worse. Have you had cervical problems, abnormal Pap smears? If so, a cervical cap might not be the best choice for you. Diaphragms and condoms and female condoms may, on the other hand, actually protect you against cervical cancer, since many experts feel this disease is linked to the sexual transmission of a virus called HPV, human papillomavirus. Are you allergic to latex? That's what condoms and diaphragms are made of. Do you have fibroids (noncancerous tumors of the uterus)? You can probably use an IUD as long as the uterine cavity is not misshapen by them. The Pill wouldn't have been an option years ago, when higher doses of estrogen sometimes caused fibroids to grow, but with today's low-dose formulations, this is no longer a problem.

Take Information Home to Read

Ask for any written information your doctor may have about the methods you're considering, or the method you have chosen. Be sure to read everything carefully, and call your doctor right away if you come across anything that makes you think you shouldn't use that contraceptive after all. No matter how carefully you and your doctor try to go over the relevant ground, sometimes things get missed, or misunderstood. Nobody's perfect. And realistically there's simply not time for every doctor to ask every patient every possible question. (See "What You Should Leave Your Doctor's Office Knowing."

Health Information to Bring to Your Doctor's Office

To help your doctor help you zero in on the best birth control method, write down the answers to the following questions (or at least think about them beforehand):

- MENSTRUAL CYCLE
    - When did your last period start?
    - How long did bleeding last?
    - How heavy was the bleeding?

- Did you have cramps? Did you take anything for them?
- How old were you when your periods started?
- Are your cycles regular or irregular?

- PAST BIRTH CONTROL USE
  - What methods have you used in the past?
  - Why did you stop using them?
  - What did you like and dislike about them?
- FERTILITY
  - Have you ever been pregnant?
  - Have you ever carried a baby to term?
  - Have you had a miscarriage?
  - Have you had an abortion?
- GENERAL HEALTH
  - How old are you?
  - Do you take any doctor-prescribed medication?
  - Do you regularly take any over-the-counter medication?
  - Do you have any medical conditions or health problems?

You also need to study any information you can get about how to use the method correctly. Call if there's anything you don't understand: It's better to be a bit of a pest than to make a mistake that leaves you at risk for an unintended pregnancy. Often a nurse or physician's assistant in your doctor's office can also answer questions.

What You Should Leave Your Doctor's Office Knowing

Before you leave the doctor's office—having chosen a contraceptive method—be sure that you know the following:

- How to use you birth control correctly
- What your chances are of getting pregnant while using it
- What to do if you mess up—if you forget to take your pill before you go to bed, for example
- What the possible side effects are, and which ones you need to report to your doctor

- What is the best time of day to call the doctor's office with questions that come up after your appointment
- Who, besides your doctor, can answer your questions

21

Fertility Awareness Methods

Currently Available

- Ovulation Method
- Temperature Tracking
- Sympto-Thermal Techniques
- Rhythm

Fertility awareness methods may also be known as natural family planning and are sometimes more technically referred to as sympto-thermal techniques. Some of the most commonly used approaches to natural fertility control include charting the days of the menstrual cycle, daily temperature taking, and the observation of changes in cervical mucus. The cervical mucus technique is sometimes called the ovulation method or the Billings method. You may also have heard of the rhythm or calendar method, a term that generally refers to counting days in the menstrual cycle. These days rhythm alone is not considered by many proponents of natural methods to be an effective means of natural family planning.

It is hard to estimate with much scientific accuracy how many women rely on fertility awareness methods, either alone or in conjunction with other forms of birth control. The Ortho 1995 Annual Birth Control Study puts 9 percent of women in the categories they called rhythm and withdrawal. The 1988 National Survey of Family Growth found that about 4 percent of women said they used some type of fertility awareness; about a third of those women said they also used another form of birth control as well.

What It Is

All fertility awareness methods involve daily observation of various changes in the female body that indicate the approach of ovulation, so that intercourse can be avoided during the days of the month when a woman is most likely to get pregnant. Note: Although they may sound simple, you should not try these methods until you attend a class or get individual instruction in their use from a family planning counselor.

The same fertility awareness techniques can also be used to increase your chances of conception when you *do want to have a baby.*

How It Works

At different times during the menstrual cycle certain relatively predictable changes occur that, if carefully followed, can alert couples that it's time to avoid sex if they don't want to risk conception.

Cervical Mucus Method. During fertile times of the month the cervical mucus becomes more copious and may be seen and felt as a liquid discharge from the vagina. This clear, slippery feeling fluid (which at times can be stretched from thumb to finger) helps to nourish sperm and is a consistency that helps the sperm make their way up the reproductive tract to the egg. Even if you can't actually see any mucus during your fertile days, your vaginal opening and lips may feel slightly wet or slippery.

To keep tabs on your cervical mucus, you have to get into the habit of checking at least once a day (even every time you go to the bathroom). See if you can collect any discharge from the vaginal opening on a finger or some toilet paper. Note how much there is, if any, and its consistency.

During the time of month that a woman is *not* fertile, the cervical mucus tends to be scant, stickier, and less "stretchable." It is more likely to stay in or near the cervix, serving as a physical barrier that is hard for sperm to penetrate. During this nonfertile time you may feel "dryer" and have no visible vaginal discharge. These descriptions are general: your cervical mucus, and the changes it goes through may be different, since there is quite a bit of normal variation from woman to woman.

To be safest, all penis-to-vagina contact should be avoided (or, if you want to have sex, use a contraceptive) when the "fertile" mucus is present—and for several days after it is no longer detectable. Ovulation usually occurs around the time of month that the "fertile"mucus stops being produced (within a day or two before or after). The egg only lives for about a day if it is not fertilized, but sperm have been shown to live for as long as a week in the female reproductive tract (although they probably more typically survive about three days). Therefore some instructors advise avoiding sex as soon as any of the fertile-type cervical mucus (or a wet feeling) appears. Because menstrual blood could obscure the very early changes in the cervical mucus, especially if you have long periods, you may also be advised that it's not absolutely safe to have sex during your period.

Some vaginal infections, including yeast and sexually transmitted diseases such as trichomoniasis, can cause a vaginal discharge. It can be hard for someone without medical training to distinguish these abnormal types of discharge from the normal changes in cervical mucus.

There are also normal and natural discharges from the vagina during and after sex that can make it more difficult to distinguish cyclical changes in the cervical mucus. For this reason some proponents of this method recommend that you only have sex every other day after your period ends, on the theory that this will make it easier to distinguish sex-related discharges from cervical mucus.

Temperature Method. Your temperature when you first wake up in the morning, before you get out of bed (or do anything active in bed), is known as your basal temperature. Generally your basal temperature will go up and down at certain predictable times during the menstrual cycle.

In order to use basal temperature as an indicator of fertility, you take your temperature first thing every morning and mark the result on a chart. (A special "basal" thermometer can make it easier to detect the relatively small cyclical changes in temperature.) Normally your temperature will drop slightly just before ovulation, then rise a half degree or more for several days in a row afterward. Your temperature will probably stay elevated until your period begins, then it will fall to the original level and stay there until it drops again just before ovulation the next month. If your temperature doesn't rise, you may not have ovulated that month. If your temperature remains elevated and bleeding does not occur, you may be pregnant. Because of individual variations, it can take several menstrual cycles before you get the hang of what your cycle tends to look like on a temperature chart. As you can see on the sample basal temperature-tracking chart on the opposite page, this isn't a matter of straight, simple ups and downs.

One important limitation of temperature charting is that it cannot always predict ovulation far enough in advance. If, for example, you happen to have sex the night *before* your temperature drops, live sperm could still be in the uterus and tubes when you ovulate a day or so later, and be able to fertilize the egg. Also your basal temperature can be thrown off its usual course by a number of life's common disruptions, including illness, lack of sleep, stress, and travel.

Sympto-thermal Techniques. Women using what is sometimes referred to as the sympto-thermal method may be taught to use some combination of the above strategies and learn to note, as well, additional menstrual cycle "symptoms," such as the midcycle pain that can occur with ovulation and the breast tenderness that often precedes menstruation. Using different approaches together can increase the effectiveness of natural family planning—and can also add up to quite a bit of record keeping. Some women find all the tracking and charting cumbersome; for others it soon becomes a familiar part of the daily routine, and a reasonable trade-off for drug-and device- free contraception.

Rhythm. Typically the rhythm or calendar method depends on abstaining from sex during a woman's probable fertile days based only on counting the days of the menstrual cycle. Typically ovulation occurs on day 14, plus or minus a day or two, from the onset of your last period. (More precisely it occurs about fourteen days *before* your next period starts.) The egg, once released, lives about one day. Sperm, as we've noted, can generally survive for about three days in the female reproductive tract

Therefore if all goes according to schedule, you should be able to avoid conception if you don't have sex from about day 9 (counting backward two days from day 14, in case ovulation comes early, then three more to compensate for sperm's life span) to about day 16 (day 14 plus two in case of late ovulation). Unprotected sex would of course be most risky right around midcycle.

One of the significant limitations of rhythm is that many women have irregular cycles, and most have them at least some of the time. This method works best if you chart several menstrual cycles before you start to rely on rhythm for contraception, so that you get an idea of how long and how regular your periods tend to be.

Withdrawal. Withdrawal, also called coitus interruptus, involves removing the penis from the vagina before the man ejaculates. It is not considered to be an effective contraceptive by many proponents of natural family planning.

Probably the biggest problem with withdrawal is that it takes extreme (some might say superhuman) control for a man to pull out of the vagina while on the verge of a climax. It may be hard for the young or sexually inexperienced to know when ejaculation is impending. Having to remove the penis before orgasm may make sex less enjoyable, for one or both partners. Even if the man does remove his penis in time, he may not get far enough away, and sperm may fall on his partner's external genitals and thereby gain access to her vagina. In addition there is the possibility that there could be sperm in the pre-ejaculate (drops of fluid that are discharged from the penis before a man comes), particularly if you have sex more than once within a few hours. The chance of pregnancy from pre-ejaculate is probably quite low, but theoretically it could happen.

How Effective It Is

It's hard to know exactly how many women get pregnant while using fertility awareness methods, for a number of reasons. For one thing, as you have seen, this method isn't a single means of birth control, but several different techniques—which can be used alone or in combination. (Some people also combine fertility awareness techniques with other types of birth control, such as condoms, during fertile days.) Also the effectiveness of the "natural" techniques depends both on how carefully and consistently a couple uses them and, perhaps even more importantly, on *how consistently they abstain from sex when they know they're likely to conceive*.

And finally, there are simply not as many well-done scientific studies on most of these methods as there are for contraceptives such as birth control pills. There was one recent study, published in the *New England Journal of Medicine*, that looked at exactly when during the menstrual cycle sex was most likely to result in a pregnancy. Interestingly, virtually all conceptions occurred when couples had sex during the five days *before* ovulation, or on the estimated day of ovulation itself. After ovulation occurred the chances of pregnancy were remote.

From the numbers that are available it is clear that effectiveness varies widely. On average, however, those who depend on fertility awareness methods tend to have relatively high pregnancy rates: Typically, according to *Contraceptive Technology*, about twenty women out of one hundred will get pregnant in a year, not much higher than the eighteen per one hundred who might get pregnant using a diaphragm. If you are young and fertile and tend to have sex frequently, your risk may be higher. And if one hundred women were to use one or a combination of natural methods to the absolute best of their ability for one year, the pregnancy rate could range from as low as 1 percent to about 9 percent. Realistically, however, such low pregnancy rates could be expected only from the most highly motivated and consistently careful of couples.

How Much It Costs

These methods cost next to nothing to use. Basal thermometers (which are sensitive to very small changes in body temperature) are widely available at pharmacies for about ten dollars.

The Advantages of This Method

Fertility control methods can be used by couples who, for religious or personal reasons, wish to avoid "artificial" forms of birth control.

These methods do not involve the use of any drugs or devices (except, if you chart your temperature, a thermometer).

These methods do not affect a woman's menstrual cycle or hormones.

Fertility awareness techniques can be used along with other methods—such as barrier contraceptives like condoms and diaphragms—to further decrease the risk of unplanned pregnancy.

The techniques of fertility awareness can also help couples recognize their most fertile times, so they can more easily conceive a child when they want to.

Learning these methods can help women become generally more knowledgeable about and comfortable with their bodies and their menstrual cycles.

The Disadvantages of This Method

It takes motivation, record keeping, and attention to detail to successfully practice the techniques of natural family planning.

It can take several months of charting the body's natural fluctuations (temperature, cervical mucus, or a combination of the two) before most women can use these methods with confidence.

It can be hard to observe the changes in cervical mucus accurately. It can be difficult for someone who is not a trained professional to distinguish normal cervical mucus from some types of vaginal infections. In addition, changes in the cervical mucus may be obscured by the vaginal discharge that occurs during and after sex, and also by menstrual blood.

These methods can interfere with the spontaneity of sex. It takes self-control for couples to avoid having sex during fertile times of the month. Intercourse must be avoided for a significant portion of each month for these methods to be most effective. (Exactly how long depends largely on your cycle's length and regularity.)

These methods provide no protection against sexually transmitted diseases—which include everything from the very common herpes and chlamydia to HIV, the incurable virus that causes AIDS.

Reversibility

All natural methods are immediately and completely reversible. As we have said, many of the same strategies that are useful in helping couples avoid pregnancy can also be used to help them conceive when they are ready to have a child.

Safety and Side Effects

Natural family planning techniques have no direct side effects and are often described as being entirely safe. However, one "risk" that women should consider carefully if they decide to use this approach is that the risk of unplanned pregnancy is higher than with many other methods.

Who Is A Good Candidate for This Method

Couples who cannot or choose not to use any other type of birth control.

Women with regular, predictable periods.

Women who are willing and able consistently to carry out the self-testing necessary to zero in on the time of ovulation.

Couples who have a high level of self-control.

Couples who have sex relatively infrequently (once or twice a month, for example), since they may find it less of a problem to adapt to timed periods of abstinence.

Women over forty, whose fertility is lower, as long as their periods are still regular and predictable.

Who is Not A Good Candidate for This Method

Women with irregular, unpredictable periods (which can be a sign that ovulation is also irregular and unpredictable) may find it difficult to use these techniques with confidence.

Young, highly fertile women, since they are more likely to have failures with this method, particularly if they have sex frequently (more than twice a week), which increases the odds that there will be live sperm in their reproductive tracts at the time of ovulation.

Couples who find it hard to refrain from vaginal intercourse during "unsafe" times of the month.

NOTE: To work best, fertility awareness techniques require counseling. *Don't try to figure them out on your own, or put them to practice after simply reading about them here*. For more information:

- A local family planning clinic (such as Planned Parenthood) may have written information and counselors who can help women learn how to monitor their cyclic changes.
- Many hospitals (particularly Catholic hospitals) have information available or hold classes to teach the techniques of fertility awareness.
- Contact Family of the Americas for information about the ovulation method. (See appendix for their address and phone number.)
- Look for books devoted to this topic at a library or bookstore. (See appendix for one example.)
- Talk to your doctor.

22

Condoms

Currently Available

Dozens of types of condoms are widely available without a prescription at pharmacies, convenience stores, supermarkets, and so on. Common brand names include Ramses, Lady Protex, and Sheik (all from Schmid); Lifestyles (Ansell); Saxon and Circle Coin (Safetex); Trojan (Carter-Wallace). Condoms come in a variety of shapes, surface textures, and colors, lubricated and nonlubricated, with and without spermicide.

According to the Ortho 1995 Annual Birth Control Study the condom is now the third most popular form of birth control in this country, ranking just below sterilization and the Pill. Currently about 19 percent of women age fifteen to fifty report that their partners use condoms. More than one in three (34 percent) young, unmarried women reported condom use. Almost half (46 percent) use condoms along with another method (such as the Pill) to protect themselves against sexually transmitted diseases, particularly HIV, the virus that causes AIDS.

What It Is

A thin, stretchy sheath about two inches wide and six inches long, designed to be worn over the penis during sex. Condoms form a physical barrier between penis and vagina and also hold sperm after ejaculation so that it cannot travel into the woman's reproductive tract to fertilize an egg.

The vast majority of condoms are made of latex, a form of natural rubber. Condoms made of lamb intestine are often referred to as skin or natural-membrane condoms. There is also one new brand (Avanti, Schmid Laboratories; FDA approved in 1994) of condom that is made of polyurethane, the same material as the female condom.

How It Works

Condoms come rolled up, in small individual packets. To use one, unroll it (being sure you have it right side out, so that it unrolls easily) onto the man's penis after he has an erection. The condom should reach all the way down to the base of the penis near the man's public hair. It must be put on before the penis has *any* contact with the

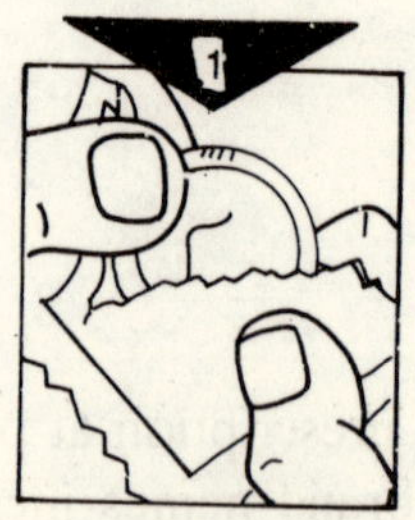

BEFORE SEX
Use a new condom every time you have sex—before foreplay, before penis gets anywhere near any body opening. (To avoid exposure to any body fluid that can carry infection.) Handle condom gently.

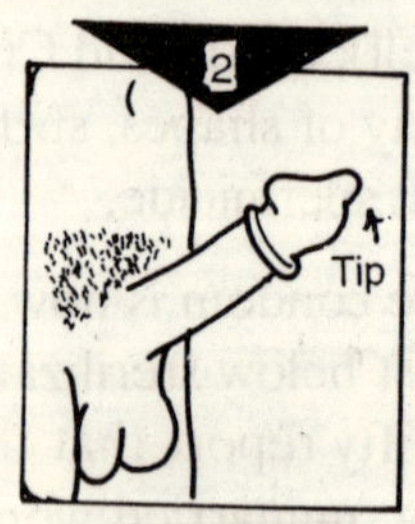

Put condom on as soon as penis is hard. Be sure rolled-up ring is on the outside. And leave space at tip to hold semen when you come.

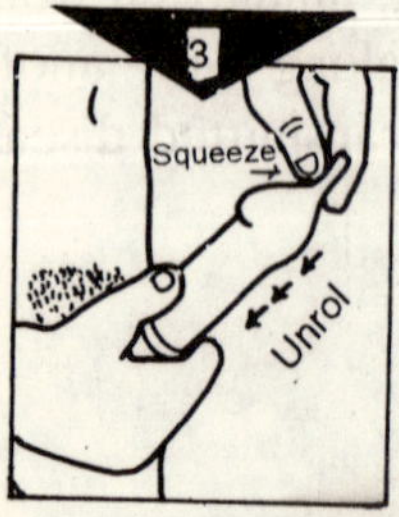

Squeeze tip gently so no air is trapped inside. Hold tip while you unroll condom . . . all the way down to the hair. If condom doesn't unroll, it's on wrong. Throw it away. Start over with a new one.

Putting on a Condom

woman's genital area. It is possible that the small amount of fluid that comes out of the penis before ejaculation (climax) could contain sperm, particularly if you have sex more than once within a short period of time. If the condom has a plain tip instead of a reservoir tip, squeeze out the air and leave about a half inch at the head of the penis to hold the semen. If the man has not been circumcised, the foreskin should be pulled back to put the condom on.

The penis should be withdrawn from the vagina as soon as the man ejaculates (reaches his climax or comes), before the penis starts to soften. The condom should be held close to the base of the penis while this is done. Once the penis is well away from the woman's genitals, the condom should be taken off carefully, without spilling any of the semen.

Condoms are designed to be used once, then thrown away. If you have sex again, no matter how soon, you should use a new condom. If you put a condom on the tip of the penis to unroll it, and discover it is inside out, you should throw that one away and use another one. Wrap used condoms in toilet paper or facial tissue before you throw them away so that no one else will end up touching the secretions. (Many people flush used condoms down the toilet, but it's not good for the sewage system).

How Effective It Is

Used correctly, condoms are a very effective method of birth control. If latex condoms were used exactly according to directions every time a couple had sex, the failure rate would probably be as low as 3 percent—surprisingly close to that of the Pill. Average pregnancy rates are significantly higher: Out of one hundred typical users, about twelve will get pregnant. That's a bit more effective than the diaphragm, quite a bit less effective than the Pill, and vastly more effective than no method at all; 85 percent of couples who use no type of contraception can expect to get pregnant in a year.

Using a condom plus a vaginal spermicide increases its effectiveness. There is not good scientific evidence to show whether condoms that come with spermicide already on them work any better at preventing pregnancy or sexually transmitted diseases than plain condoms.

About 12 million people in this country are infected with a sexually transmitted disease each year. Two-thirds of AIDS victims got the disease from having sex with an infected partner. Latex condoms provide more protection against sexually transmitted diseases (particularly HIV, the virus that causes AIDS) than any other birth control method. The only thing safer than condoms is abstaining from sex altogether. (Mutual monogamy is also safe *if you can be sure that both you and your partner are disease-free.)*

For STD protection condoms can be used during anal and oral sex, as well as for vaginal intercourse.

Condoms also provide significant protection against other STDs besides HIV. They are quite good at preventing the transmission of human papillomavirus (HPV) from the penis to the cervix. This extremely common infection causes genital warts and has been linked to cervical cancer. Condoms also provide significant protection against chlamydia and gonorrhea. Condoms are less good at preventing the spread of herpes, since this infection is spread by skin-to-skin contact, and lesions (sores) can appear on body parts not shielded by a condom (such as the buttocks, the vulva in a woman, or the scrotum in a man).

Lamb-intestine condoms have microscopic pores, smaller than sperm, but big enough to let some disease-causing germs through, and should not be used for protection against STDs. Laboratory tests on polyurethane condoms (both male and female) suggest that this material should be very good at blocking diseases, but so far there is limited information about how well it works with real people under normal circumstances.

How Much It Costs

Latex condoms generally cost about fifty cents each or less, making this one of the most inexpensive contraceptives available. If you have sex twice a week for a year, it would add up to about one hundred dollars. Sheep-intestine and polyurethane condoms cost more. If you get latex condoms from a family planning clinic or college health service, they may cost even less.

The Advantages of This Method

Condoms are widely available and don't require a prescription.

Condoms are relatively inexpensive, and you only need to buy them when you need them. (In contrast, for example, you have to take the Pill every day, even if you have sex only on weekends; and methods such as IUDs and Norplant must be paid for up front and remain active in your body whether you need contraceptive protection or not).

Condoms can be used along with other types of contraceptives (such as the Pill or an IUD) specifically for disease protection.

Condoms are a good backup to have on hand for added contraceptive protection in case you forget to take a birth control pill.

Tips For Successful Condom Use

- Don't underestimate the power of a condom: They can be almost as effective as the Pill in preventing pregnancy and they are unmatched in their ability to prevent sexually transmitted diseases—*if you use them correctly every time you have sex.*
- For an extra edge of protection, against both pregnancy and diseases, use a vaginal spermicide along with condoms. You can put a little bit in the tip of the condom before you put it on, and a little more on the outside of the condom after you put it on—or use an applicator to put extra spermicide directly into the vagina.
- Be sure the condoms you buy say on the label that they provide protection against sexually transmitted diseases. Not all condoms do (lambskin, some imported condoms), and only those that do can say so on the label.
- Put the condom on before there is any contact between penis and vagina. A small amount of fluid (possibly containing enough sperm to cause a pregnancy) comes out of the penis before ejaculation.
- For the most complete protection against STDs, use condoms during oral and anal sex, as well as for vaginal intercourse. (Condoms may be more likely to break during anal sex). If you're going to have oral sex, apply spermicide afterward. It won't hurt you but it doesn't taste good.
- Use a new condom every time. Don't try to reuse them.
- Don't use Vaseline, baby oil, skin creams or any type of oil-containing products for extra lubrication, since they can weaken latex. There are a number of condom-safe lubricants available. (K-Y jelly is one popular brand). Spermicides also work for lubrication.
- Condoms vary in length and width, in how lubricated they are (how "slippery" they feel), in surface texture (ribbed, studded, etc.), color, flavor, and more. If you or your partner don't like one kind, try others until you find one you like better.
- If the condom is too tight, it may be more likely to break; if it's too loose, it may slip off during sex.
- Keep extra condoms away from heat and light (pockets, car glove compartments, and wallets are not recommended). Open the packet just before you use it, and toss any condom that's not soft, flexible, and fresh looking.
- Be careful not to snag the condom on long fingernails, teeth, or jewelry.

- If a condom breaks or comes off during sex, wash with soap and water right away (which can reduce the risk of infection, not pregnancy). It is sometimes recommended that a woman immediately apply a vaginal spermicide in this situation. While this may reduce the number of live sperm in her reproductive tract, sperm swim fast, and some are likely to get through the cervix before you can get the spermicide in place. (Another good reason to use condoms plus spermicide to begin with). You may want to call your doctor or clinic for advice if the breakage or slip-off occurs around midcycles, when you would be likely to be ovulating. Depending on a number of factors (such as your medical history and exactly when during sex the condom actually broke), you might be a candidate for the "morning-after" pill. ("When Birth Control Fails.") If so, it must be taken within seventy-two hours.

The Disadvantages of This Method

For condoms to work, you have to use them every time you have sex.

Unlike other barrier methods, this is not a contraceptive women can use to protect themselves: The man must be a willing and active participant.

It takes discipline to use condoms correctly. You have to put them on during sex—after a man has an erection—and take them off again while the penis is still hard after ejaculation.

Some people find it embarrassing to buy condoms at a store, or to talk about using them with a new sexual partner.

Men frequently complain that they don't like the way condoms feel—that they don't transmit body warmth, for example, and that they cut down on sensation. Then again, millions of couples have found ways to enjoy sex with condoms in spite of these limitations. And as more and more women start to insist on condom use to protect themselves from STDs, more and more men are likely to decide that sex with a condom beats no sex at all.

Reversibility

Condoms are immediately and completely reversible: Any time you don't use one, you could get pregnant.

Safety and Side Effects

Condoms are very safe and have virtually no side effects. They don't affect sperm production or the semen itself in a man or the menstrual cycle or hormone levels in a woman.

A small number of people are allergic to latex and will be unable to use condoms (or diaphragms or cervical caps) made out of this material. For them a polyurethane condom (male or female) might be a good alternative.

Who Is A Good Candidate for This Method

Women whose partners are willing to use condoms.

Couples with good self-control and the discipline to use condoms every time they have sex.

People who are at risk for sexually transmitted diseases.

Who Is Not A Good Candidate for This Method

Women whose partners won't use condoms.

People who are sensitive to latex.

Safety and Side Effects

Condoms are very safe and have virtually no side effects. They don't affect production of the semen itself in a man or the menstrual cycle or hormone levels in a woman.

A small number of people are allergic to latex and will be unable to use condoms (or diaphragms or cervical caps) made out of this material. For them a polyurethane condom (male or female) might be a good alternative.

Who is A Good Candidate for This Method

Women whose partners are willing to use condoms

Couples with good self control and the discipline to use condoms every time they have sex

People who are at risk for sexually transmitted diseases

Who is Not A Good Candidate for This Method

Women whose partners won't use condoms

People who are sensitive to latex

23

Female Condoms

Currently Available

Reality female condom (Female Health Company, Wisconsin Pharmacal). The female condom was approved by the FDA in 1993 and has been widely available in this country since 1994. Because this method is still relatively new, we are unable to reliably report how many women are using it.

What It Is

A thin, colorless, flexible tube of polyurethane, about 6 inches long and 2 inches wide, that is open at one end and closed at the other. There are rings at each end, both of which are softer, thinner, and more flexible than the ring that forms the rim of a diaphragm.

The female condom is designed to be worn by the woman, lining the vagina. This method is intended to provide protection against both pregnancy and sexually transmitted diseases. Unlike a diaphragm, the female condom is used alone, without additional spermicide; also unlike a diaphragm, the female condom is "one size fits all."

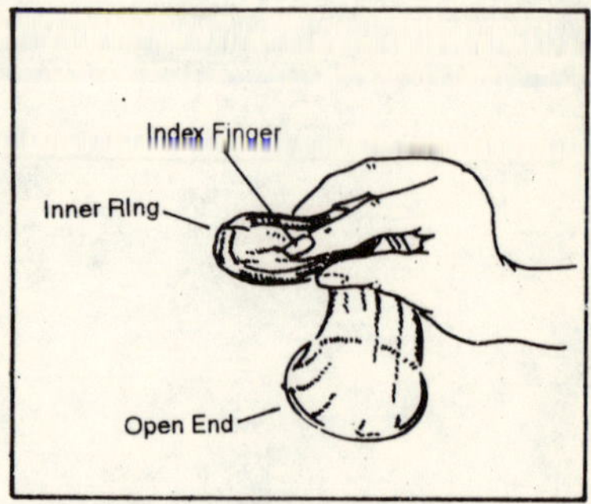

1. Iner ring is squeezed for insertion

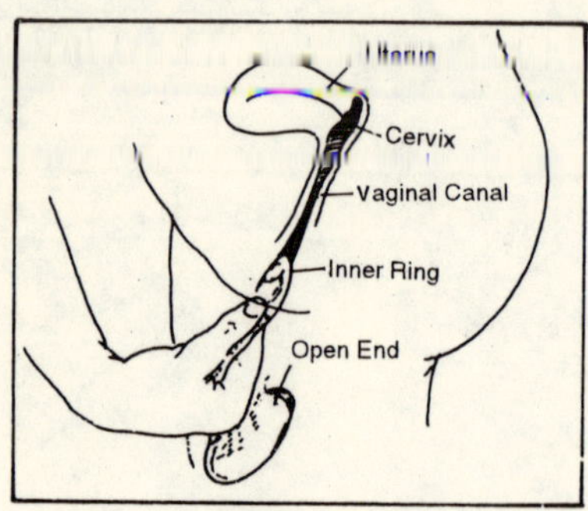

2. Sheath is inserted, similarly to a tampon

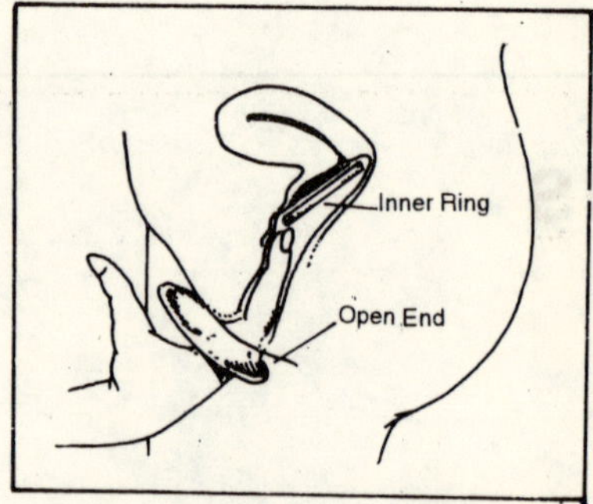

3. Inner ring is pushed up as far as it can go with index finger

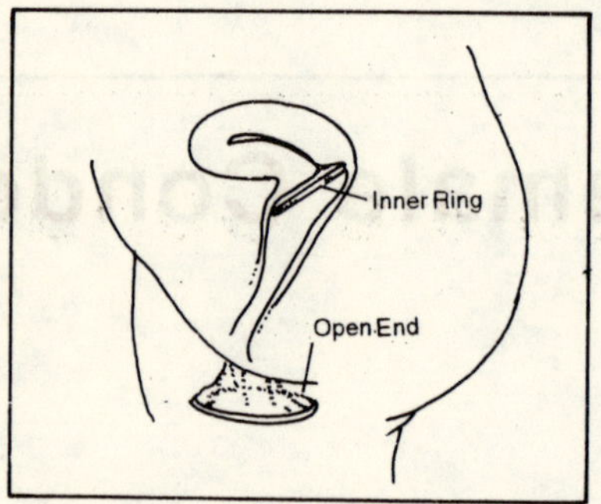

4. In place

Inserting the Female Condom

How It Works

The female condom is a physical barrier between a woman's vagina and a man's penis. It catches and holds the semen that is released from the penis so that the sperm cannot enter the woman's reproductive tract and fertilize an egg.

Female condoms, like their male counterparts, are available without a prescription at drugstores, supermarkets, and so on. They come individually wrapped in plastic pouches that are bigger than the tiny packets that hold male condoms, since Reality does not come rolled up like a male condom. Like male condoms, female condoms are designed to be used one time only, then thrown away.

The female condom looks like a stretched-out version of male condoms, except for the soft rings at each end, which help hold it in place. The inner ring is held close to the cervix by the public bone, the way a diaphragm is; the outer ring simply rests outside the body, covering the vaginal lips (the labia).

You can put in the female condom standing up, squatting, or lying down. Although technically it can be inserted as long as eight hours ahead of time, according to the package insert, most women will probably find it more comfortable to insert, the condom just before they have sex, instead of walking around with it in. Wash your hands before inserting the female condom. To put it in, hold the vaginal lips apart with one hand, and use the other hand to squeeze the inner ring flat and slide the condom into the vagina. Be sure you put the *closed* end (with the smaller ring) into the vagina. Keep pushing the inner ring with your finger until it is all the way up the vagina, past the public bone. When it's in right, the inner ring will be hooked behind your pubic bone and the outer ring will be lying against your vaginal lips on your pubic hair. (About an inch of the tube will usually be visible, too). The condom must lie straight, not twisted, in the vagina.

After the man ejaculates, pinch the outer ring closed and twist the condom to keep the semen inside. Then gently pull the condom out, wrap it in tissues or toilet paper, and throw it away. Don't flush it down the toilet (it's bad for the sewage system), and don't try to wash it out and use it again. If you have sex again, you need to use a new condom.

While you don't have to take the female condom out immediately after the man ejaculates, as you do with a male condom, it is still a good idea to remove it relatively quickly, and definitely before you stand up—so semen doesn't leak. (The reason the penis and male condom have to be withdrawn *immediately* is that the condom won't fit tightly as the penis softens, and semen could seep out).

How Effective It Is

In the six-month clinical trials of the female condom, pregnancy rates were about 13 percent, which—doubled—would make the annual pregnancy rate about 26 percent. Those are the statistics you will see on the package insert (and is a higher pregnancy rate than is typically cited for male condoms or diaphragms), but some experts think female condoms actually work better than this number suggests. Failures tend to taper off after people have used a method for a while and gotten the hang of it, so accidental pregnancies in the second six months should be lower than during the first six months (bringing the yearly total down). But because female condoms have not been around that long, and because studies on other barrier methods were done differently, it's hard to predict how the pregnancy rate for the female condom will compare with that of other barrier methods in the long run. After more data are collected, it is possible that the FDA will allow changes in the labeling with regard to pregnancy rate.

Barrier methods in general have higher pregnancy rates than methods such as the Pill or IUDs. Based on limited data, the female condom seems to have a slightly higher pregnancy rate than male condoms, and about the same pregnancy rate as diaphragms, cervical caps, and sponges (which are no longer available in this country as of this writing). Women who use no method at all have about an 85 percent chance of getting pregnant in a year.

Like the male condom, the female condom should provide significant protection against sexually transmitted diseases. In laboratory testing, the polyurethane female condom did not let any STD-causing germs through, including viruses, the tiniest of these invaders. However, there are, so far, limited scientific data available about STD protection when the female condom is used in normal circumstances by regular human beings. Because it covers more body area than a diaphragm or cervical cap, and doesn't allow any contact between a woman and the man's semen, this method may prove to provide more protection against at least some types of STDs (including HIV, the virus that causes AIDS) than those barrier methods.

How Much It Costs

Reality condoms cost a lot more than male condoms—about seven or eight dollars for a box of three. They may cost less if you get them from a family planning clinic or college health service.

The Advantages of This Method

Unlike male condoms, this method is used by women, giving them a new means of control over their sexual health.

The female condom can be inserted into the vagina before sex, so some people find that it interrupts sex less than male condoms (which can only be put on after a man has an erection).

Men (and women) may find they like the softer, looser feel of the female condom more than the tight male condom.

People who are allergic to latex (the material most condoms, diaphragms, and cervical caps are made of) can use this method.

The female condom should provide significant protection against many types of sexually transmitted diseases, including HIV, the virus that causes AIDS.

The Disadvantages of This Method

The female condom is new and odd-looking, which may make some people reluctant to give it a try. (Think back, though, to the first time you saw a male condom; they are not exactly elegant, either).

Like all barrier methods, female condoms only work—protecting you against pregnancy and sexually transmitted diseases—when you use them. You have to have one ready and waiting— in your purse, in your bedside-table drawer--when you are ready to have sex.

Because of the possibility of human error, barrier methods in general have higher pregnancy rates than methods such as IUDs, the Pill, or Norplant.

You are likely to be more aware of the female condom during sex (especially the first couple of times you use it) than you would be with other methods, including other barrier methods. For example you and your partner will probably be aware of the outer ring shifting as you move. Both men and women have complained of pubic irritation.

Reversibility

This method is immediately reversible. If you don't use it, even once, you could get pregnant.

Tips For Using Female Condoms

- This is a relatively new method that people may not be familiar with. Be sure to read the instructions that come in every box (and have your partner read them, too, so that he knows what to expect) before trying to use the female condom for the first time.
- Getting the condom in and out can be a little tricky at first. It might be a good idea to practice a few times by yourself so that you don't give up in frustration or embarrassment the first time you try to use it with your partner. (Throw the "practice" condom away because it will have come in contact with your vaginal secretions.)
- It's a good idea to hold the man's penis and guide it into the condom. That way you can be sure the penis is inside the condom (not next to it), and that the condom's outer ring doesn't get pushed into the vagina.
- You can use extra lubricant with the condom if the man feels as if it's sticking to or "riding" his penis during sex. (Female condoms come with a small bottle

of extra lubricant). The lubricant can be put either on the condom or on the penis.

- If the condom "squeaks" or feels like it's rubbing either partner, try adding a few drops of lubricant or moving into a slightly different position.
- Use extra lubricant on the outer ring if it feels as if it might be pushed inside the vagina during sex. If the outer ring does go into the vagina, the package insert recommends that you stop, remove the condom, and put in a new one before continuing.
- Don't try to use a male condom and a female condom at the same time: According to the instructions they may stick together.
- Be careful not to snag and tear the condom on teeth, fingernails, or jewelry.
- If you keep extra condoms on hand and don't have sex for a while, be sure to check the expiration date on the box before you start to use them again.
- All of the above will probably get a lot easier once you and your partner have tried this new method a few times.
- If you have any problems with or questions about the female condom, ask your doctor or someone at your family planning clinic or health service, or call the free phone number on the Reality female condom box: 1-800-274-6601.

Safety and Side Effects

This method is very safe. It has no effect on anything inside a woman's body—it doesn't affect your menstrual cycle or your natural hormones. It doesn't require the use of any additional chemicals (such as spermicide), as the cervical cap and diaphragm do. There is nothing about this method that would be expected to have any effect on a fetus if you did accidentally conceive while using it. Polyurethane has not been reported to cause allergic reactions.

Who Is A Good Candidate for This Method

Women (or couples) who want to protect themselves against pregnancy and sexually transmitted diseases.

Women who are willing to use the female condom every time they have sex.

Women who can afford this relatively expensive barrier method.

Couples who find they enjoy using this method more than male condoms.

Women who have sex infrequently and don't want, or need, the everyday protection of methods such as the Pill or an IUD.

Who Is Not A Good Candidate for This Method

Women who would find it hard to use female condoms correctly and consistently. A big part of consistent use is having your contraceptive where you are when you need it. Also key: a willing partner.

Those who find the condom's appearance unappealing.

Men or women who experience rubbing or irritation from the outer ring.

24

Vaginal Spermicides

Currently Available

Vaginal spermicides are widely available without a prescription at drugstores, supermarkets, and so on. They come in a variety of forms, including

- Foams (popular brands include Emko, Delfin, Koromex)
- Creams and jellies (such as Ortho Gynol II, Koromex, Conceptrol)
- "Inserts", or suppositories (such as Semicid and Encare)
- "Film" (vaginal contraceptive film, or VCF, is not as widely available as the other forms of spermicide)
- Spermicide-saturated sponges (the Today vaginal contraceptive sponge was discontinued in 1995 due to manufacturing problems and as of this writing is no longer available in the United States)

Most of the spermicides available in this country contain the sperm-immobilizing ingredient nonoxynol-9. A few contain a very similar chemical called octoxynol. Some spermicides are designed to be used alone, other packages indicate that the product is meant to be used with a diaphragm or cervical cap, but there is not really much difference between them.

Approximately 3 per cent of women rely on spermicides for birth control, according to the Ortho 1995 Annual Birth Control Study.

What It Is

Unlike other barrier methods, spermicides (used alone) provide a chemical barrier, rather than a physical one, against conception. (Vaginal sponges did offer both, when they were available). Spermicides are designed to be placed in the vagina to kill the sperm before they can reach and fertilize a woman's egg.

How It Works

Spermicides are chemical "surfactants." Much the way surfactants in your laundry detergent dissolve greasy stains, the surfactants in spermicide dissolve the fatty components in the membrane that covers the sperm, which kills them.

Whatever type of spermicide you choose (foam, cream, etc.), it must be inserted into the vagina, as close to the cervix as possible, before any contact with the man's penis. Foams, creams, and jellies start to work as soon as you put them in, and stay active for about an hour. Inserts and vaginal films take about ten to fifteen minutes after you put them in to melt and disperse before they become fully effective. (Encare may cause a feeling of warmth in the vagina as it foams and expands). Since time and other specifics do vary, be sure to read the package and follow the instructions before you use any type of spermicide.

If you have sex more than once, or if you wait more than an hour before having sex, most package instructions say that you should put in another dose of spermicide. If you are using the spermicide with a diaphragm the instructions usually tell you to insert another dose into the vagina (without removing the diaphragm) if you have sex again before it's time to take the diaphragm out. If you are using your spermicide with a cervical cap the instructions usually say additional spermicide is not required, although it certainly can't hurt, and may help maintain effectiveness. If these recommendations sound a bit vague, they are. Spermicides simply haven't been subjected to the kind of intense, long-term scientific scrutiny that newer, more "hightech" prescription methods such as the Pill, the ParaGard IUD, Norplant, and Depo-Provera have undergone. The recommendations that do exist are based on limited scientific data—combined of course with large doses of the experts' common sense and decades of practical experience.

How Effective It Is

Used alone, vaginal spermicides tend to have high failure rates. Of one hundred typical users, about twenty-one are likely to get pregnant during one year of use. If spermicides were used according to directions every time a couple had sex, the pregnancy rate would probably be substantially lower—more on the order of six pregnancies in those one hundred couples. That's still twice as many as for perfect use of condoms, but much fewer than if no method is used: If those one hundred couples used no method for a year, eighty-five of them would be expected to get pregnant.

These numbers, it should be noted, are estimates, unlike the more precisely known failure rates quoted for methods such as the Pill, Norplant, IUDs, and Depo-Provera—or even condoms—all of which, as explained above, have been studied more extensively and in more scientifically exacting ways than have spermicides alone.

Spermicides used together with condoms are more effective than either method used alone.

As for sexually transmitted diseases, spermicides have been shown to be able to kill the germs that cause most common STDs in a test tube. Although it's likely that they do provide some measure of protection in real-life use, it is impossible to say exactly how much. Unlike condoms, spermicides are not allowed by the FDA to claim protection against STDs on their packages and labels. There is also a complicating factor here: There have been studies showing that very frequent, prolonged use of spermicide (the original studies were done on prostitutes in Africa) seem to be associated with sores on the walls of the vagina—which could theoretically end up making women more vulnerable to infection, rather than less. While this probably does not happen with the amounts of spermicide most people use most of the time, until more studies are done, it is impossible to say for sure exactly how much spermicide it might take to have this effect.

How Much It Costs

As with condoms, how much this method costs will depend on how often you have sex. Although prices vary, depending on the type of spermicide you buy and where you buy it, you will probably end up spending about twenty-five cents per dose. That would add up to about twenty-five dollars a year, or less, if you had sex an average of twice a week and only used spermicides.

The Advantages of This Method

Spermicides are widely available at supermarkets, drugstores, and convenience stores.

They require no prescription and no doctor visit for a woman to be able to use them.

They are very safe. They do not affect menstruation or a woman's natural hormone cycle.

They are relatively inexpensive.

Your can buy as much or as little as you need, and only when you need birth control.

Unlike with condoms, a woman can use this method without a man's cooperation, although he will probably be aware that you are using it.

The Disadvantages of This Method

As with all barrier methods, you have to use spermicides every time you have sex. However, you can apply spermicide to the vagina before intercourse, so it doesn't interrupt lovemaking the way condoms can.

Spermicides used alone tend to have high failure rates—higher than with other barrier methods that provide a physical barrier between egg and sperm, and significantly higher than with methods such as the Pill and IUD.

The chemicals in spermicides can cause irritation in one or both partners.

Spermicides alone provide much less protection against STDs than condoms.

Reversibility

Spermicides are immediately reversible. If you use them, you are protected against pregnancy. If you don't use them, even once, you could get pregnant.

Safety and Side Effects

Spermicides are very safe and are not known to have any systemic effects. There may be some absorption into the body (there have been reports of Encare causing a soapy taste in some women's mouths, for example), but this has never been shown to be harmful in any way.

Sometimes spermicides cause irritation. You or your partner might notice an itching or burning sensation on your genitals. Sometimes people think that they have a urinary tract infection or a vaginal infection and it takes them a while to figure out that the spermicide is causing their symptoms. If one brand or formulation bothers you or your partner, it's possible that a different one might not.

A number of years ago there was a widely publicized report suggesting a possible link between spermicide use early in pregnancy and birth defects. This report has been criticized for its design and analysis—it was a retrospective study that relied on women's memories of having bought spermicide in the six months before they got pregnant. Today the consensus of expert opinion is that there does not appear to be a cause-and-effect link between spermicides and birth defects. If you are worried about this possibility, discuss it with your doctor.

As discussed above, there is the possibility that prolonged use of large amounts of spermicide might cause sores in the vagina and increase the risk of transmission of some types of sexually transmitted diseases. This is probably not a problem when spermicides are used as most people do—one, possibly two doses, several times a week.

Tips For Effective Spermicide Use

- As with all barrier methods, spermicides work only when you use them.
- Always insert the spermicide as close to the cervix as possible.
- Wash your hands before inserting a spermicide. If there is an inserter, also wash that with soap and water after you use it.
- Be sure to give the spermicide time to foam or melt, if necessary, before you have sex. How long you have to wait after insertion varies from type to type: Be sure to read the package insert of the kind you buy.
- Apply more spermicide if you wait more than an hour to have sex.
- Apply more spermicide if you have sex more than once.
- Keep an extra package handy so that you don't run out unexpectedly.
- If one form or brand of spermicide is irritating to either you or your partner, try a different one. If it still bothers you, you will probably have to consider other contraceptive options.
- Don't douche after sex for at least six hours, or you may lower the spermicide's effectiveness. Douching does not work as a contraceptive. Most doctors con-

sider it unnecessary at best. If you feel better after douching, talk to your doctor about the safest way to do so.

Who Is A Good Candidate for This Method

Women who have the discipline to use spermicides consistently and correctly every time they have sex. Spermicides can be kept on hand even if you regularly use another method. They can be used along with methods such as fertility awareness or condoms for an extra measure of protection against an unplanned pregnancy. You can also use spermicide as a backup if you miss more than one birth control pill.

Who Is Not A Good Candidate for This Method

Women who would find it difficult to use spermicides every time they have sex. It takes discipline to use this and other barrier methods.

Because of the typically high failure rate, women who have medical reasons that could make a pregnancy dangerous should seriously consider more effective methods.

25

Diaphragms

Currently Available

- Koro-Flex Arcing Spring Diaphragm (London International U.S. Holdings)
- Koromex Coil Spring Diaphragm (London International U.S. Holdings)
- All-Flex Arcing Spring Diaphragm (Ortho-McNeil Pharmaceutical)
- Ortho Coil Spring Diaphragm (Ortho-McNeil Pharmaceutical)

As of 1995 about 1.7 million (3 percent) women in this country used a diaphragm, according to the Ortho 1995 Annual Birth Control Study. This method is most likely to be used by married women between the ages of thirty and thirty-nine. Two-thirds of the women who use this method have done so for at least five years.

What It Is

A soft natural rubber (latex) device, shaped like a shallow bowl, with a firm but bendable rim. The rim is designed to fold so that the diaphragm can be slipped into the vagina. As soon as you let go, the diaphragm opens to cover the cervix.

Diaphragms are designed to be used with spermicide. Before insertion, about a teaspoon of spermicide is placed into the bowl of the diaphragm and a small additional amount is spread around the rim.

Diaphragms are available by prescription only, since they must be sized to each woman individually by a doctor or health professional in order to fit—and therefore work—properly.

How It Works

The diaphragm works in two ways. First, it serves as a physical barrier that covers the cervix to keep sperm from entering the uterus and tubes, where they might fertilize an egg. Second, the bowl of the diaphragm holds the spermicide and keeps it concentrated around the cervix.

Unlike a condom, which must be put on a man's erect penis during sex, a woman can put in her diaphragm before—even hours before—having sex. To insert it, hold the diaphragm rim up, squeeze the rim flat with one hand, hold the vaginal lips open with your other hand and slip the diaphragm into the vagina. (Wash your hands first.) Push the front of the rim with one finger until it slips into place behind the public bone. When it's in the right place, the spermicide-filled dome of the diaphragm will be covering the cervix. You should be able to feel the cervix through the rubber.

After you have sex, you must leave the diaphragm in place for six hours to give the spermicide time to kill all the sperm. To remove the diaphragm, hook a finger under the rim and gently pull it out. If you have sex again before the six hours is up, just insert more spermicide into your vagina, leaving the diaphragm in place. Start counting the hours to removal from the last time you have sex.

After removing the diaphragm wash it with mild soap and water. Be sure to rinse it well, since soap could damage the rubber if left on the diaphragm for a long time. Dry it thoroughly and put it back in its case to protect it from damage. Over time your diaphragm may become stained or discolored. As long as there are no holes in it (you should check for holes every time you use it), the diaphragm will still work.

How Effective It Is

Diaphragms, like natural methods of family planning and other barrier methods, are frequently subject to human error. If one hundred women used their diaphragms perfectly (according to directions every time you have sex) for one year, about six of those women would get pregnant. That's a higher pregnancy rate than would be

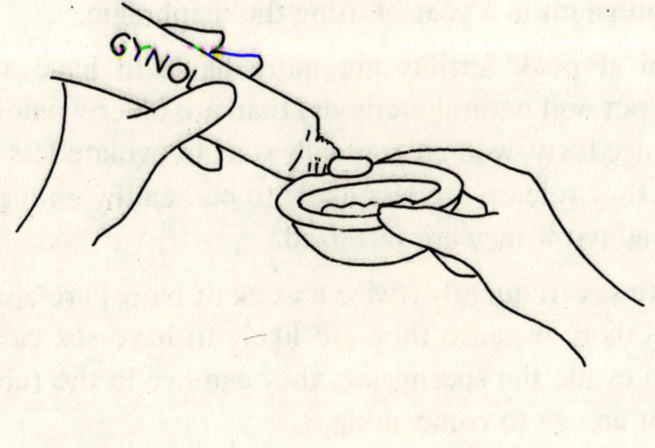

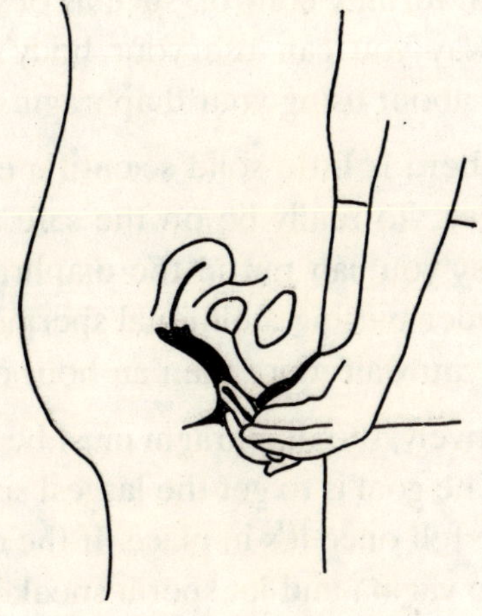

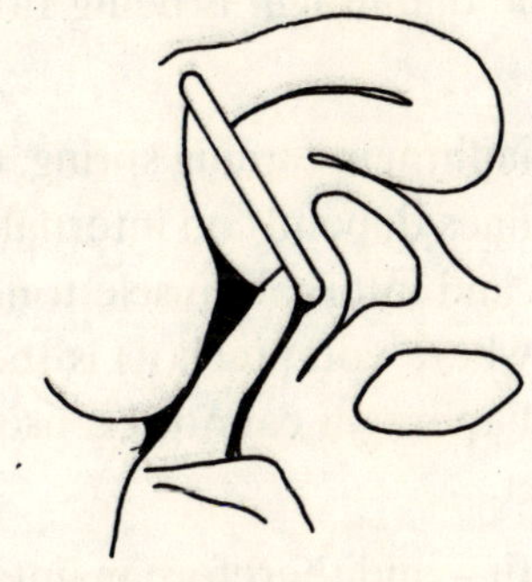

Inserting the Diaphragm

expected with perfect use of condoms. More typically about eighteen out of one hundred women become pregnant in a year of using the diaphragm.

Younger women at peak fertility are more likely to have a failure with this method (and other barrier and natural methods) than are older women whose fertility is declining. After about age forty, women gradually start to ovulate less frequently, and as time goes by, the eggs they release are less likely to be healthy enough to be fertilized, or to make a healthy embryo if they are fertilized.

Women who have sex frequently (twice a week or more) are also at higher risk of pregnancy with this method, because they are likely to have sex close to the time of ovulation. If any sperm evade the spermicide, they can live in the tubes and uterus for several days, waiting for an egg to come along.

It can be helpful for women who use this and other barrier methods to be familiar with the techniques of natural fertility control, such as observing the natural changes in your cervical mucus. That way you can use your body's signs of peak fertility as a reminder to be extra diligent about using your diaphragm exactly right.

Perhaps surprisingly, there is little solid scientific evidence to show exactly how long spermicide remains active. To really be on the safe side, then—and even though package instructions often say you can put in the diaphragm up to six hours ahead of time—you may want to consider putting additional spermicide into the vagina (without taking the diaphragm out) if you wait more than an hour or so to have sex.

In order to work effectively, the diaphragm must be fitted properly by a doctor or trained health professional. The goal is to get the largest size possible that is not uncomfortable to insert and can't be felt once it's in place. If the diaphragm is too small, it may move around too much in the vagina and let sperm sneak by; if it's too big, it may press against the urethra (the tube through which urine exits the body) and possibly contribute to urinary tract infections. Although it can be hard to do so, it's important to try to relax as much as possible while the diaphragm is being fitted, otherwise you might end up with a too-small size.

The type of spring on the diaphragm (arcing spring, coil spring) is largely a matter of personal preference, but sometimes depends on internal physical characteristics (such as the size and position of organs and internal muscle tone). Some experts feel that an arcing rim (which compresses anywhere you pinch it) is the easiest for women to put in correctly. However, this type of diaphragm cannot be used with an inserter—a plastic holder—which some women prefer.

To ensure the best possible fit—and therefore maintain the highest possible effectiveness while you use this method—your doctor should check your diaphragm's size if you gain or lose more than about ten pounds, if you have vaginal or pelvic surgery, or if you have a baby or an abortion. Even if none of the above apply, it's a good idea to double-check the fit when you see your doctor for your routine exams.

How Much It Costs

A diaphragm costs about twenty dollars and, as long as it doesn't develop any holes, can be used for about two or three years. Spermicide costs about twenty-five cents per use. In considering the total cost of this method, remember that you have to see a doctor to have it sized correctly in the first place and that you should have the fit checked yearly. (Simple size rechecks shouldn't add much, if anything, to the cost a regular gynecologic checkup.)

The Advantages of This Method

Safety and immediate reversibility rank high on this method's list of advantages.

This method (unlike condoms) is entirely within a woman's control: You can put it in well before sex and be protected against pregnancy.

As with all barrier methods, you only need to use this method when you have sex. (Unlike the Pill, Which you have to take every day, even if your partner's on a business trip for two weeks; or Norplant, which stays put until you take it out, whether or not you even have a partner).

Studies have shown that using a diaphragm plus spermicide can cut approximately in half a woman's risk of sexually transmitted diseases and pelvic inflammatory disease, a serious infection that can result from undetected infections. Diaphragm users have also been reported to have a lower risk of cervical abnormalities and cervical cancer. In a test tube, spermicides have been shown to kill the germs that cause many sexually transmitted diseases, including gonorrhea, herpes, and HIV However, studies (on prostitutes) have shown that very frequent use of unusually large quantities of spermicides may result in sores in the vagina, which theoretically might increase the risk of HIV infection. Further studies under more normal circumstances are needed to clarify the relationship between HIV susceptibility and spermicide use.

The Disadvantages of This Method

Probably the biggest disadvantage of this method (and one that is true of all barrier methods) is that you have to be very motivated to use the diaphragm correctly and consistently every time you have sex.

The diaphragm is available by prescription only. You must go to a private doctor or family planning clinic or college health service to have the device individually fitted: Diaphragms come in a variety of sizes and with one of two types of springs in the rim (which makes a difference in how they fold for insertion).

Some women find it hard to insert the diaphragm—the process can be uncomfortable, or the device can fail to slip into proper position. Coil-spring diaphragms can be used with an inserter, which some women find makes them easier to put in. Sometimes getting it in isn't the problem, but getting it out is. Squatting (or sitting on the toilet) and straining (pushing) as if for a bowel movement can help move the diaphragm lower in the pelvis and make it easier to remove.

Some who try it complain that the diaphragm is messy and interferes with the spontaneity of sex. Certainly this method isn't for everyone. But couples who have used diaphragms successfully usually find ways around the potential problems and find that the drawbacks are outweighed by the advantages. As we've noted, a diaphragm doesn't interfere with sex if you put it in well beforehand. (If you don't end up using it, you can just take it out again.) Some couples find it perfectly acceptable to incorporate diaphragm insertion into foreplay itself, as one does with condoms. If you find that the spermicide makes everything too slippery, maybe you're using too much—or maybe another brand, or a cream formulation instead of a jelly would work better for you.

Reversibility

The diaphragm is an immediately reversible method of birth control. If you use it, you use it, you are protected against pregnancy; if you don't, you aren't. It's totally up to you.

Safety and Side Effects

The diaphragm is generally considered to be a very safe method of birth control.

About ten years ago there was an unsettling study that suggested spermicides might cause birth defects if accidentally used early in pregnancy. Since then other studies have not supported this report, and most experts are now convinced that spermicides do not cause birth defects. The original report has come under a great deal of criticism for the way it was designed and for the conclusions it reached.

A small percentage of the population will have an allergic reaction to latex, or natural rubber, which will mean they can't use this contraceptive. (These are the same people who also won't be able to use latex condoms or cervical caps.)

Some people are sensitive to spermicides, which would cause itching or burning when they're used. This sensitivity can occur in either partner. There is also, as mentioned above, the currently unresolved question of whether using very large amounts of spermicide over long periods of time might cause sores or ulcers on the walls of the vagina and the cervix.

There have been reports suggesting that diaphragms might increase the risk of urinary tract infections, especially if they are not fitted properly. Call your doctor if you have the following symptoms, which can indicate an infection: pain when you urinate, blood in the urine, fever, feeling like you have to urinate all the time even if nothing comes out. Most urinary tract infections are easily treated and respond quickly to prescription antibiotics.

Tips for Successful Diaphragm Use

Putting the diaphragm in and taking it out can take a bit of getting used to. Be sure you are comfortable doing this and that you know how to check that it's in the proper position *before you leave the doctor's office or clinic*. Once at home, try inserting and removing the diaphragm in different positions (standing with one foot on a chair, squatting, lying on your back) to see which you find easiest and most comfortable.

- Wash your hands before putting the diaphragm in or taking it out. Don't get petroleum jelly (Vaseline) or any skin creams containing oils on the diaphragm, since this can weaken the rubber.
- For the diaphragm to work, it must be in the right place: covering your cervix. After you put it in, you should be able to feel your cervix (a firm protrusion at the top of the vagina) through the rubber dome of the diaphragm.
- Try changing positions during sex if you or your partner can feel the rim of the diaphragm.
- If you're worried that this method will make sex less spontaneous, remember that you can put the diaphragm in ahead of time.
- If the diaphragm is too slippery to grasp and squeeze flat, you may be putting too much spermicide around the rim.
- It's a good idea to keep extra spermicide (and even an extra diaphragm) on hand in case you need it on short notice.
- Use more spermicide if you have sex again before it's time to take the diaphragm out. Don't move the diaphragm. Leave it where it is and simply put the spermicide into the vagina.

- Package instructions usually say to insert more spermicide into the vagina if you wait longer than six hours to have sex. To be on the safe side (since nobody really knows exactly how long spermicides remain active), you might want to put in the extra dose if only an hour or so has gone by.
- Check the diaphragm when you wash it to make sure there aren't any rips, holes, or worn-out-looking areas. If the diaphragm starts to look worn, replace it.

There is also some concern about the possibility that the diaphragm might increase a woman's risk of toxic shock syndrome (TSS), which most people have heard about in connection with tampon use. There have been a few cases reported in the literature in which this apparently has happened, and the possibility is mentioned in the package insert. Although toxic shock is rare, it can be deadly. For this reason anyone who has had toxic shock in the past should not use this method. It is possible that leaving the diaphragm in the vagina for long periods of time might increase the risk of TSS. You are supposed to leave the diaphragm in for six hours after the last time you have sex—but after that, to be on the safe side, you should try to take it out as soon as possible. The package instructions say you shouldn't leave it in for more than twentyfour hours. The symptoms of toxic shock can include a sudden high fever, vomiting, diarrhea, faintness, and a sunburnlike rash. Joints and muscles may ache and the eyes may redden. If you suddenly spike a fever and have even one of the other symptoms, take out the diaphragm immediately and call your doctor.

Who Is A Good Candidate for This Method

Highly motivated women who are willing to use this method every time they have sex.

Older women in stable relationships. Because fertility is past its peak, the risk of unintended pregnancy is lower for these women. Long-standing couples may also have the time and motivation to work out some of the kinks of diaphragm use, such as when and where to put it in and take it out.

Women whose lives are predictable enough, or who are good enough at planning ahead, to know that the diaphragm will be where they are when they need it.

Women who have medical reasons for not using the Pill or an IUD.

Women who are familiar with this method can also use it (instead of condoms) as a backup if they forget to take a birth control pill.

Who Is Not A Good Candidate for This Method

Couples who would find it hard to use their diaphragm every time they wanted to have sex.

Women who are highly fertile and have sex frequently, since this and other barrier and natural methods may have too high a failure rate.

Women who are not comfortable touching their genitals.

Women who have recurring urinary tract infections when they use the diaphragm.

Any woman who has had toxic shock syndrome in the past.

26

Cervical Caps

Currently Available

The Prentif Cavity-Rim cervical cap was approved by the FDA for use in the United States in 1988. It is manufactured by Lamberts, Ltd., in Luton, England, and distributed in the United States by Cervical Cap Ltd., in Los Gatos, California.

Far fewer women (and doctors) in this country know about cervical caps than its barrier-contraceptive cousin, the diaphragm. The device is more popular in England and is also available in European countries, including France and Switzerland, as well as in Canada and Australia.

What It Is

A thimble-shaped device made of natural latex rubber (the same material as most diaphragms and condoms) that is designed to fit closely over a woman's cervix. The cup part of the cap is soft and flexible, the rim is firm, and about one and one-half inches wide. There is a groove on the inside rim of the cap that creates a seal against the cervix and helps hold it in place.

Like diaphragms, cervical caps come in different sizes, and you need to go to a doctor or family planning clinic to have one fitted for you.

Cervical caps are used with spermicide. You fill the cup about one-third full before inserting it.

How It Works

The cervical cap works in two ways. It is a physical barrier that fits closely over the cervix, preventing sperm from entering. It also works as a holder for spermicide, keeping this additional chemical barrier concentrated close to the cervix, where it's most needed. Because it must be precisely the right size to hug the cervix, not all women can be properly fitted with a cervical cap. The fit must be more exact than with a diaphragm.

To insert the cap, squeeze the rim flat with one hand while holding your vaginal lips apart with your other hand. (Washing your hands first). Gently push the cap, rim

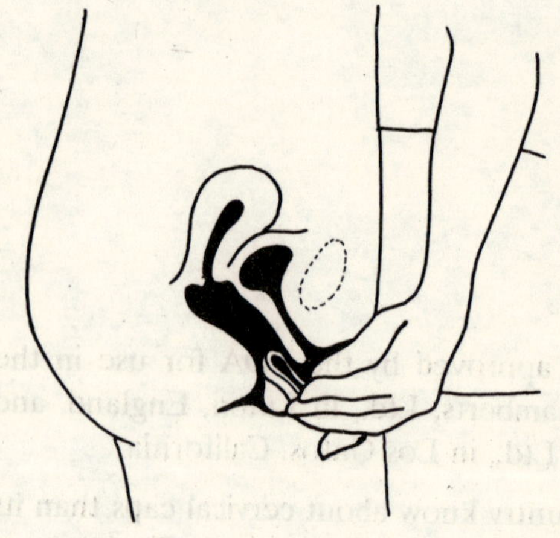

Hold cap pinching the sides together. Reach back to place cap on the cervix.

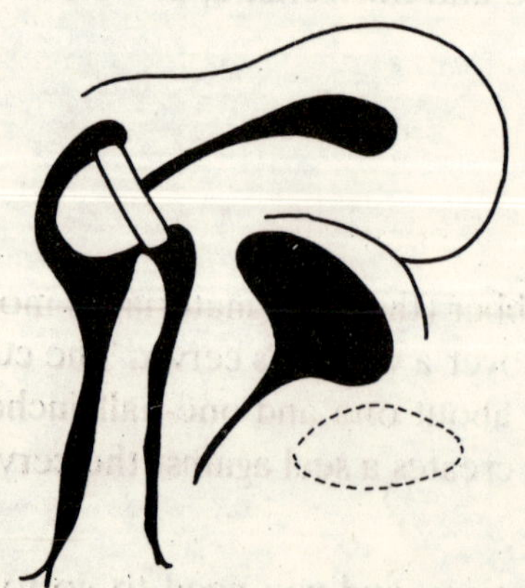

Check placement of the cap with index and middle finger. The cervix should be completely covered by the cap. The dome should feel soft with some dimpling.

(Cervical Cap Ltd.)

Inserting the Cervical Cap

end first, into the vagina and as far up as it can go, until it covers the cervix. If the cap doesn't slip into place, you can either try to push it over the cervix with your fingers or you can take it out and start over again. When the cap is in right, it completely covers the cervix—run a finger around the rim to check. It also won't come off easily if you push it with a finger, or when the penis bumps it during sex. You should also be able to feel the cervix through the rubber dome fo the cap. The dome won't be tight against the cervix, since there has to be a little space to hold the spermicide and any secretions from the cervix.

You must leave the cap in place for eight hours after the last time you have sex to be sure that any sperm that manage to get into the cap have been killed by the spermicide. The longest you should leave the cap in is forty-eight hours, according to the package instructions, because of a possible risk of toxic shock syndrome.

The cervical cap instructions say you don't have to put in more spermicide if you have sex more than once. However, there's a lack of good scientific data showing precisely how long spermicide actually stays active in the cap, so it certainly can't hurt—and may well give you an extra edge of protection—if you do use more. Insert extra spermicide into the vagina without moving (or removing) the cap.

To get the cap off the cervix when it's time to remove it, use a finger to gently break the seal between cap and cervix, then pull the cap down and out of the vagina. Squatting and bearing down (as if pushing out a bowel movement) can help make the cap easier to reach. Wash the cap in mild soap and warm water, and rinse and dry it well before you put it away.

How Effective It is

It is hard to be precise about how well the cap prevents pregnancy, in part because it has not been used, or studied, all that much in this country and in part because effectiveness seems to vary greatly from woman to woman, depending on variables such as how well the cap fits and how diligently she uses it.

According to *Contraceptive Technology,* among women who have not had children, about eighteen out of every one hundred would typically get pregnant during a year of using the cervical cap. Used correctly every time, the cap's failure rate in this group drops to about nine in one hundred. The cap may be significantly less effective in women who have had children: Typical failure rates are listed at 36 percent; perfect use at 26 percent. The Prentif Cap's package insert says it's between 82.6 and 93.6 percent effective, "depending on consistency of use."

There really isn't a lot of good scientific evidence that directly compares barrier methods to one another. Scientifically it's not considered accurate to compare the results of separate studies, since researchers don't all use the same rules and standards; instead the contraceptives should be compared directly in the same study so that the same conditions would apply to each method.

Used consistently and correctly, male latex condoms plus vaginal spermicide are generally considered to be more effective in preventing pregnancy than the cervical cap plus spermicide. Nonbarrier contraceptives such as Norplant and IUDs have higher "typical" effectiveness ratings, because once they're in place, they work. Remember, many, if not most, failures with barrier methods occur primarily because *don't* use them correctly and consistently.

The cervical cap and spermicide will provide some protection against sexually transmitted diseases, although it's hard to know exactly how much. It would be logical to expect the cap to provide less protection (at least against certain diseases) than the male or female condom, since condoms prevent direct contact between penis and vagina, while the cap only covers the cervix.

How Much It Costs

Cervical caps cost about the same as diaphragms—around twenty dollars for the device alone. Because you have to go to a clinic or private doctor to have the cap properly fitted and to learn how to put it in and take it out, you will need to take into account this cost too. As long as the cap is in good shape, it can be used for up to three years before you replace it.

Cervical caps are used with spermicide. This additional cost (about twenty-five cents per use) will depend on how frequently you have sex. Twice a week would add up to about twenty-five dollars a year.

The Advantages of This Method

The cervical cap can be used by a woman and does not require a man's cooperation.

This method can be put in hours ahead of time if you want to, so it doesn't interrupt sex.

The cervical cap can be left in place for up to forty-eight hours, although it sometimes causes an odor problem with prolonged use. During that time you can have sex as many times as you want. (With all other barrier methods you have to either apply more spermicide or use another condom each time you have sex. However, even for this method, adding spermicide each time you have sex could give you an extra edge of effectiveness).

This method has no known bodywide effects. It does not change a woman's hormone levels, and it does not affect menstruation or fertility.

The Disadvantages of This Method

Although it does provide some protection, the cervical cap does not defend against sexually transmitted diseases as well as latex male condoms do.

As with the diaphragm, you have to go to a doctor to have the cap fitted correctly.

It can be difficult to find a doctor who is knowledgeable about fitting caps and how to use them.

Some women find the cervical cap difficult to put in and take out (more so than the diaphragm).

This method cannot be used during menstruation. It also cannot be used by a woman who has a vaginal or cervical infection or bleeding, or an abnormal Pap smear result, or until six weeks after a woman has a baby, a miscarriage, or an abortion.

Some men report that they can feel the cervical cap during sex.

This method has a higher failure rate than many other kinds of contraceptives.

Reversibility

The cervical cap is immediately and completely reversible. Any time you don't use it, you could get pregnant.

Safety and Side Effects

The cervical cap is generally a very safe contraceptive that causes no systemic side effects.

Some women have abnormal Pap smear results (microscopic changes in cervical cells) when they use the cap. You will have to switch to another method of birth control if this condition persists. When you get a cap, your doctor will probably ask you to come in for a Pap smear after about three months, just to be sure everything's okay.

A small number of women and their partners are sensitive to latex and will be unable to use this method. Some people are also sensitive or allergic to spermicides.

There has been some suggestion that using a cervical cap might increase a woman's risk of toxic shock syndrome, a rare but potentially fatal illness. (This is the same type of toxic shock that has been reported with tampon use). It is not known how much a cap user's risk is increased, or if in fact it is actually increased at all. To be on the safe side, the cap is approved for use for no longer than forty-eight hours, on the theory that prolonged use increases risk. Any woman using a cervical cap (or diaphragm or tampons) should be familiar with the symptoms of toxic shock: sudden high fever; fainting or dizziness; sore throat; muscle aches and pains; red, sunburnlike rash. Remove the cap and call your doctor immediately if these symptoms occur.

Who is a Good Candidate for this Method

Women who will be able to use this method consistently and correctly every time they have sex.

Women who can get the hang of putting the cap in and taking it out.

This method might work well for women who have sex mostly on the weekends, since you can leave it in place for up to forty-eight hours.

A cervical cap might be a good choice for older, slightly less fertile women in stable relationships who don't want to use methods such as the Pill or an IUD and who would feel comfortable working through the "learning period" necessary with this method.

Who is not a Good Candidate for this Method

Women who can't get a proper fit with the cap.

Women who have trouble putting the cap in and taking it out. Many find this harder to do than with a diaphragm. If you can't use it easily, a cap is unlikely to be a good choice for you.

Women who are sensitive to spermicides (they cause burning or itching) or to latex, or whose partners are sensitive to spermicides or latex.

Women who develop cervical problems (i.e., abnormal Pap smear results) when they use the cap.

Any woman who has had toxic shock syndrome.

Any woman who has undiagnosed vaginal bleeding or a vaginal or cervical infection, until it is treated and clears up.

Any woman who has had a baby, a miscarriage, or an abortion in the past six weeks, because the shape and/or size of the cervix may change.

Women who have medical reasons that would make a pregnancy dangerous. Such women should carefully consider whether any barrier method is the best possible choice for them, because of their relatively high failure rates. If it is the best option, study up on the fertility awareness methods discussed in chapter 4; using them in conjunction with a barrier method may help you decrease the risk of accidental pregnancy.

Tips for Successful Cervical Cap Use

- Be sure you are comfortable with inserting and removing the cap and that you know how to check that it's in proper position *before you leave you clinic or doctor's office.*
- Once you get home, try putting the cap in and taking it out in different positions (squatting, standing with one leg on a chair, lying on your back) to see which is easiest for you.
- The package instructions suggest using a backup method (such as condoms) for about a week at home while you and your partner get used to the new method. Check the cap before and after sex to make sure it stays in position. If it comes off, you may need a different size: don't use the cap any more until you see your doctor again. (If you find out after sex that the cap has been dislodged, you may want to check with your doctor about whether emergency contraception might be indicated in your particular situation).
- Always wash your hands before inserting the cap; and don't let anything oil-based (including petroleum jelly, baby oil, many skin creams, and some vagina medications) touch it. Oil makes latex deteriorate quickly.
- Before you put it in, check the cap for holes or tears.
- Always use spermicide along with your cervical cap. Although the method doesn't require it, you may want to apply more spermicide for extra protection before repeating sex.
- don't' forget to take the cervical cap out. It is likely to cause a bad odor, and may possibly increase your risk of toxic shock syndrome, if you don't.
- Have condoms available to use during menstruation.
- Remember, for this method (or any barrier contraceptive) to work, you have to use it every time you have sex.

27

The Earlier Trimesters

This chapter discusses emotional changes and sexuality during the first and second trimesters, common physical changes of pregnancy, fetal growth and development, and nutrition information.

Emotions

Pregnancy is a time of self-reflection and growth for most people, both as individuals and as couples. Most authorities call it stressful and a time of change in identity and maturation. There appears to be a commonalty to the process of adjusting to the reality of parenthood, although each person reacts in different degrees, depending on his or her background. You may find it reassuring to know that other couples have many of the same feelings and concerns that you have. Let's take a closer look at the process of becoming parents.

The Mother's Feelings

In general, women report that they have more mood swings, are more open about their feelings, are more aware of the cycle of life, and seem to have increased emotional reactions to events. Probably the most common feeling at this time is ambivalence about being pregnant, no matter if the pregnancy was planned or not. "Is this really the best time to be pregnant?" "I wonder if I can really be a good mother?" "Will the baby love me?" "What will happen to my career?" It takes time to accept this new, very special, and exciting reality—you're going to be a mother.

Toward the end of the first trimester, pregnant women usually become more introspective, remembering the relationship they had with their own mothers. This a step towards developing their own mothering roles.

By the second trimester, most women have accepted the reality of their pregnancy. The thrill of hearing the baby's heartbeat and feeling him move in the uterus verifies his existence, and you may find yourself imagining your baby's personality, sex, and physical characteristics. The baby is now recognized as a separate person. At the same time, a woman often needs more affection and reassurance from her mate, and she may become more dependent on him and increasingly concerned over his safety.

The Father's Feelings

Fathers, too, must accept the reality of the coming event. ambivalence is a common emotion—you are facing possible financial changes, the reality of "settling down," and the responsibilities of parenthood. Most men are proud of their virility. An increase in emotions usually occurs, with which some men are more comfortable than others. You may feel rivalry or resentment toward the baby if your mate is more introverted and giving you less attention. You may feel left out.

You will have reactions similar to those of the mother during the second trimester. When your feel your baby move, the emotions and realities of fatherhood begin. Your idea of the baby's looks, sex, and personality develops, although most men tend to imagine an older child rather than an infant. It is no wonder that at such an emotional time fathers often experience increased creativity, some at work, some at home, and others in artistic outlets.

As a pregnant couple you are sharing many emotions, doubts, needs, and joys. Because you are unique, your reactions to pregnancy may differ from one another and other couples. It is important to be aware of and to talk about your needs and to offer each other support and love.

Sexual Relations

Most women need more tenderness, reassurance, and intimacy from their partner during pregnancy. This emotional nourishment is important—the mother-to-be thrives on it, and it is necessary for her to develop maternal love.

Sexual relations during pregnancy can help meet this need for attention and affection. Oftentimes, though, pregnancy alters a couple's sexual desires and intimacy and can cause concern or anxiety unless they understand the reasons for the change. There are no data to support a general theory about when couples feel more or less sexual desire. The phases of pregnancy can affect each woman in a different way. Some couples experience a decline in sexual desires and frequency of intercourse, others feel a new surge of interest.

Generally, however, there are some factors during the first trimester that can influence sexual desires, and it is helpful for couples to realize that some of these may alter their sexual relationship.

1. There is a relief that contraception is no longer necessary. This freedom can have a positive effect on a sexual relationship. Some couples feel relaxed and comfortable during the months in which they are trying to conceive, whereas others with infertility problems can be frustrated and tense. Unless it was unplanned, most couples feel a great deal of satisfaction once conception has been confirmed.

2. After conception, hormonal changes begin to affect the woman's body. Many women are overwhelmingly fatigued during the first trimester, and all they want to do is sleep. Nausea and vomiting can affect a woman's sexual desires, and real or imagined fears of miscarriage may make couples avoid intercourse of orgasm. The physician can advise couples about whether intercourse and/or orgasm would be a threat to the pregnancy. In most cases it is not. A changing body with enlarged, sensitive breasts may create pride in some women and enhance their sense of sexuality. Thus the woman's changing body and the fact that she is now carrying a baby may enhance the couple's sexual life.

Many couples report an increase in sexual desire and lovemaking during the second trimester. Nausea, fatigue, and the fear of miscarriage are usually over. The uterus is enlarging but is not yet much of an obstacle. Although the baby is beginning to move, it is not yet kicking vigorously.

Many women feel that the second trimester is the time of greatest physical comfort during pregnancy. An enlarged uterus and movements of the baby help make the pregnancy a reality to both mother and father. Together these can enhance a couple's lovemaking.

Common Physical Changes of Pregnancy

In addition to emotional changes during pregnancy, there are many physical ones, which may be easier to tolerate if you understand the reasons for their occurrence.

Women vary in their reactions to them. Some of you will be bothered by going to the bathroom quite frequently and others will simply accept it as part of having a baby.

The following is a list of the more common changes or complaints of pregnancy and suggestions to help make them more tolerable.

Nausea and vomiting: Morning sickness

Cause: Believed to be caused by adaptation of the body to pregnancy, allowing the stomach to become empty, and changes in carbohydrate metabolism; aversions to certain foods and odors can also cause nausea. Usually only occurs during the first trimester.

Suggestions: Eat smaller amounts of food five to six times per day.

Eat dry toast or crackers before rising in the morning. If these conditions are severe, your doctor may prescribe medication.

Breast Changes

1. Breast sensitivity or tenderness (tingling, throbbing sensation); enlargement of breasts; prominence of veins.

   Cause: Hormonal changes and increased blood supply to the breasts.

   Suggestions: Wear a bra that fits well and gives good support.

2. Darkening of areola (dark skin around nipple).

   Cause: Increased hormones during pregnancy: disappears following pregnancy.

3. Colostrum: Precursor to milk; can be manually expressed by third month of pregnancy.

   Cause: hormonal changes.

   Suggestions: None.

Constipation

Cause: Increased pressure of the uterus causes crowding of the digestive organs.

Suggestions: Drink a glass of warm water before breakfast.

Watch your diet. Drink plenty of fluids, especially water and juices. Eat adequate roughage—bran, whole wheat products, fruits, and vegetables. Try an occasional natural laxative such as figs, prune juice, raisins.

Get adequate exercise.

Use only doctor-recommended stool softeners and laxatives and only if diet doesn't help.

Hemorrhoids: Varicose veins of the rectal area.

Cause: Pressure of the uterus on the rectum interferes with venous return: aggravated by constipation.

Suggestions: Watch your diet to avoid constipation.

Apply ice packs, or doctor-recommended medication.

Heartburn: Mild to severe "burning" behind the sternum or breastbone.

Cause: The pregnancy hormone, progesterone, may cause relaxation of the stomach's cardiac sphincter, allowing the stomach's contents to spill back into the esophagus.

Suggestions: Eat smaller amounts more frequently. Eat slowly. Sleep with your head elevated on several pillows. Avoid spicy foods.

Use only doctor-recommended alkaline medication, and only if these suggestions don't help.

Do not use baking soda because the sodium content is too high.

Varicose veins: Enlarged veins whose walls have thinned and stretched.

Cause: Progesterone may contributed to the problem by causing muscle relaxation. Return of blood from the legs is poor because of uterine pressure on blood vessels.

Suggestions: Avoid prolonged standing if at all possible. When standing, shift your weight from one foot to the other. Elevate one leg on a stool if possible.

Lie with your legs elevated higher than your heart or hips so that the blood pooling in your legs is relieved. Try to do this for five minutes every hour. Do the sand-digging exercise.

Avoid constricting clothing: tight pants, knee-high hose, girdles. Elevate the end of your bed or sleep on your left side with your legs elevated on several pillows.

If your doctor recommends it, put on support hose first thing in the morning.

Do not sit with your felt or legs crossed.

Calf Cramps

Cause: pressure of the uterus on the nerves supplying the lower extremities; fatigue, chilling, or tension in legs; an imbalance in the amount of calcium and phosphorus in your body (too much phosphorus).

Suggestions: Avoid pointing your toes like a ballet dancer.

If the calf cramps, pull your toes up toward your face and stretch the calf muscle or stand on the cramped leg and bend your knee while keeping your heel on the floor.

Your doctor may prescribe pills to increase your calcium intake.

Edema: Swelling of hands, feet, sometimes face.

Cause: Retention of fluids in the body.

Suggestions: Sleep on your left side with legs elevated; rest frequently in this position during the day.

Headaches are possible because edema can occur in your head, which cannot enlarge because of the skull bones. However, if headaches continue, call your doctor.

Use moderation in your salt intake. Do not eliminate salt completely. Avoid those foods high in sodium: carbonated beverages salad dressings, and the like. Use salt when your cook, but watch your use of table salt.

Increase your fluid consumption.

Follow the suggestions for varicose veins.

Call your doctor if swelling is extreme. Fluid retention, especially in your face and hands, can be a symptom of toxemia.

Backache: Universal Complaint of Pregnancy

Cause: Increased sway in your lower back caused by the weight of the enlarging uterus; relaxation of the pelvic joints because of the ovarian hormone, relation; stress on the uterosacral ligaments which attach to the back of the uterus and the sacrum, or backbone. Stress on these ligaments increases as the baby's size increases.

Suggestions: Make an effort to maintain good posture at all times. Wear shoes with a slight heel and good support. Avoid highheeled shoes; they increase the curve in your spine.

If backache occurs, do pelvic tilts and have your mate rub your back.

Skin Changes

1. *Striae Gravidarum:* Stretch marks on the abdomen, breasts, hips, buttocks, and thighs.

Cause: Breakdown of skin tissue as it stretches to accommodate the growing fetus.

Suggestions: Stretch marks cannot be prevented of removed once they appear. From their original red appearance they will fade to a less noticeable silvery white mark. If they itch, a body lotion may be soothing.

2. *Linea Nigra:* Dark line from umbilicus (navel) to the genital area.

Cause: Hormonal changes causing increased pigmentation of the skin.

Suggestions: None. The line usually remains after pregnancy, although it is not as noticeable.

3. *Chloasma:* "Mask of pregnancy"—irregular blotches of brown on a woman's face.

Cause: Hormonal changes.

Suggestions: It will disappear after pregnancy, and can be camouflaged with makeup.

Urinary Frequency

Cause: Pressure of the uterus on the bladder, especially noticeable during the first and third trimesters.

Suggestions: Relief in the first trimester occurs as your uterus continues to grow up and out of the pelvis, relieving pressure on the bladder. Relief in the last trimester occurs only with delivery of your baby.

Round ligament pain: Sharp, sudden pain in the groin area.

Cause: Sudden movement which puts pressure on the already greatly stretched ligaments supporting the uterus.

Suggestions: Move carefully and avoid sudden movements. Turn over carefully when you're in bed or getting up.

Bleeding Gums

Cause: Insufficient Vitamin C.

Suggestions: Eat more foods rich in Vitamin C. Be sure to brush and floss your teeth daily (see the discussion on nutrition later in this chapter).

Shortness of Breath

Cause: Expanding uterus applies upward pressure on the diaphragm, especially in the last trimester.

Suggestions: Maintain good posture. Sleep with your head elevated on pillows. Avoid lying flat on your back. This condition is alleviated as your baby moves lower in your pelvis near the end of pregnancy.

Fetal Growth and Development

Although much fetal development occurred before pregnancy was confirmed, it is included here because it is such an intriguing subject. These highlights of fetal development are thoroughly discussed and illustrated in Geraldine Flanagan's excellent book, *The First Nine Months of Life.*

Most fetal *development* occurs during the first trimester of pregnancy. Most *growth* occurs during the second and third trimesters.

Conception occurs when an egg released by the woman's ovary is *fertilized* or penetrated by a sperm from the man. The result is a single cell—the beginning of your baby.

The egg is round and much larger than the sperm, which resembles a dot with a tail, only much smaller. Only one egg is released each month by the woman's ovaries. Twenty to 500 million sperm are present in a single ejaculation of semen. Neither the egg nor the sperm can survive longer than a day or so. Thus, conception can only occur on one or two days of the woman's menstrual cycle. The sperm carries the man's genes, including the sex of the baby; the egg carries the woman's genes.

The sperm released during intercourse may pass through the cervical mucous during the proper phase of the woman's menstrual cycle. The sperm travels through the uterus into the Fallopian tube where fertilization usually occurs. The fertilized egg continues its two-or three-day journey down to the uterus. It has now become 36 cells. The fertilized egg continues to divide into many cells so that by seven days there are about 150 cells. These cells are different from one another—some are programmed to become blood, others brain tissue, and so on.

The egg implants, or "nests," no the uterine wall about one week following conception and becomes the site of the placenta. It may implant high in the uterus and remain there during pregnancy or implant low in the uterus and move up later.

The cells continue to increase—great changes are taking place day by day—so that by the end of month, the whole *embryo* has been formed. Only a quarter of an inch long, the tiny body has arm and leg buds and a head. Although a very simple organism, the embryo has eyes, ears, mouth, brain, kidneys, liver, and a blood stream. Your baby's heart began beating around the twenty-fifth day.

"By the end of the month the embryo completes the period of relatively greatest size increase and greatest physical change of a lifetime. The month old embryo is ten thousand times larger than the fertilized egg was."

By the seventh week, all the baby's internal organs are present. She is only one inch long, but her heart, liver, and kidneys are functioning. During the third month she begins to move, although the mother is probably not aware of her movements. The baby swallows amniotic fluid. She is about three inches long, weighs an ounce, and has human features.

By about six months your baby has grown to approximately a foot in length and weighs around one and one-half pounds. Her eyes open and she moves about in a quart of amniotic fluid. Her body systems and organs are still immature. During the third trimester, growth and maturation of these systems will be completed.

At the beginning of the eighth month your baby, weighing about two and a quarter pounds, is viable—that is, capable of surviving outside of the uterus—but if born at this time, would require intensive medical care.

During the last three months, some of the mother's immunities are transferred to the baby. These antibodies will help protect the baby during her first six months of life. The placenta produces gamma globulin which helps protect the baby and makes the mother more resistant to disease during this last trimester.

At birth your baby will have grown to be more than 200 million cells—all from her beginning as a single cell.

Nutrition

Nutrition has long been an unglamorous subject, yet one that is extremely important to the pregnant woman. The quality of the food you eat before and during pregnancy affects your unborn child.

Eating nutritious foods that supply the requirements your body and baby need can contribute to a healthier baby. Faulty intake reduces the available building material necessary for the development of fetal cells.

The development of sound eating habits now will carry over to the diet your offer your child once he begins to eat solids, and in general, your entire family will benefit.

Some Facts About Weight

1. "The Committee on Maternal Nutrition of the National Academy of Sciences recommends an average weight gain of 24 pounds during pregnancy. This is commensurate with a better than average course and outcome of pregnancy."
2. A weight gain of more than 40 pounds is generally discouraged.
3. During the first trimester your should gain 1 1/2 to 3 pounds.
4. During the remainder of your pregnancy you should gain a little less than 1 pound per week.

5. You should not attempt to lose weight at any time during pregnancy.

Although sources vary about the distribution of weight gain, the following is an approximate breakdown:

Fetus	7 to 8 pounds
Placent	1 pound
Fluid	2 pounds
Breast tissue	3 pounds
Uterus	2 pounds
Protein storage	4 pounds
Blood volume	4 pounds
	23 to 24 pounds

Calories and Nutrients

During pregnancy calories provide energy to build the new tissue of the placenta and fetus and to sustain the mother's body during a time when it is working overtime.

1. The 25-to-30-year-old woman, weighing 128 pounds and being 5'5" tall, requires approximately 2,000 calories per day to maintain good health.
2. During the latter half of pregnancy, the pregnant woman needs approximately 300 more calories per day than the nonpregnant woman.
3. The woman who is breast feeding (lactating) needs approximately 500 more calories per day for milk production.

A woman has an increased need for many different nutrients during pregnancy and lactation. The suggested daily requirements of the following nutrients are from the *Food and Nutrition Board, National Academy of Sciences-National Research Council Recommended Daily Dietary Allowances.*

Protein is essential for (1) production and maintenance of cells, muscles, and tissue in the baby; and (2) repair and maintenance of cells, muscles, and tissue in the mother's body.

The nonpregnant woman needs 46 grams of protein per day. The pregnant woman needs 76 grams, and the lactating woman needs 66 grams.

Iron is an essential part of hemoglobin, which enables red blood cells to carry oxygen through the mother's body and to the baby. Iron is needed for (1) fetal growth and development—the formation of fetal blood supply; (2) storage by the fetal liver for use during the first few months of life; (3) reserve for the mother following delivery; and (4) maintenance of hemoglobin levels in the increased maternal blood supply.

The nonpregnant woman needs 18 milligrams of iron daily. During pregnancy and lactation the need remains the same. Many physicians prefer that their pregnant patients have a higher intake of iron.

Your doctor will check your iron level during pregnancy by a simple blood test, which measure the amount of hemoglobin in your red blood cells. A low hemoglobin reading indicates low iron, or *anemia*.

Good sources of iron include liver, cooked dry beans, lean beef, spinach and other dark green leafy vegetables, raisins, prunes, dried peaches and apricots, and eggs.

Five milligrams of iron is supplied by 2 ounces of liver or 1 cup of beans. It is difficult to get sufficient iron from diet alone, so during pregnancy a supplement of 30 to 60 milligrams of iron daily is often recommended during the second and third trimesters.

Folic acid is a B vitamin that is essential for (1) normal growth and development of fetal cells, and (2) development of red blood cells.

The nonpregnant woman requires 400 micrograms of folic acid daily. During pregnancy the need increases to 800 micrograms, and during lactation to 600 micrograms.

Sources of folic acid include beef and chicken liver as well as dark green leafy vegetables and brewer's yeast. Because it is difficult to get sufficient folic acid from diet alone, it is usual to prescribe folic acid as a vitamin supplement during pregnancy.

Vitamin C (ascorbic acid) is essential for (1) resistance to infection; (2) formation of bones and teeth; (3) the healing process; (4) healthy gums and teeth; and (5) maintenance of cartilage, bones, muscles, and tissues.

The nonpregnant woman needs 45 milligrams of vitamin C daily. During pregnancy the need increases to 60 mg, and during lactation to 80 mg. (See also sources of ascorbic acid later in this chapter.)

Vitamin D is essential for (1) the utilization of calcium and phosphorus by bones, teeth, and blood; (2) the formation of strong bones and teeth in the fetus.

The nonpregnant woman does not require vitamin D if she is over 22, but during pregnancy and lactation she needs 400 International Units of vitamin D daily.

Vitamin D can be acquired through foods or exposure to the sun. Good sources include fortified milk, fish, egg yolks, and yeast. One quart of fortified milk daily provides the necessary vitamin D. If you have an intolerance for milk, vitamin D can be supplied by yogurt, cheese, or vitamin supplements.

Vitamin A is essential for (1) healthy skin, hair, and fingernails; (2) cell growth and development; (3) tooth formation; (4) bone growth; and (5) proper functioning of the thyroid gland.

The nonpregnant woman needs 4,000 International Units of vitamin A daily. During pregnancy the need increases to 5,000 International Units, and during lactation to 6,000 International Units.

Beef and chicken liver, sweet potato, greens, cantaloupe, and squash are good sources, as are leafy green vegetables and yellow fruits and vegetables.

Vitamin B_1(thiamine) is essential for (1) the use of carbohydrates by the body, and (2) appetite and digestion.

A nonpregnant woman requires 1 milligram of thiamine daily. During pregnancy and lactation the need increases to 1.3 milligrams because of the increased number of calories needed at this time.

Good sources of thiamine include pork, green peas, liver, oatmeal, orange juice, milk, potato, and whole wheat bread.

Vitamin B_2 (riboflavin) is essential for (1) maintenance of tissue function, (2) use of protein by the body, and (3) growth of the fetus.

The nonpregnant woman requires 1.2 milligrams of vitamin B_2 daily. During pregnancy the need increases to 1.5 milligrams, and during lactation to 1.7 milligrams.

Good sources of riboflavin include liver, milk, cottage cheese, spinach, winter squash, beef, and pork.

Vitamin K is essential for the production of prothrombin, which is necessary for blood coagulation, or clotting.

Good sources are green leafy vegetables, cauliflower, carrots, and liver.

Calcium, a mineral, is essential for (1) the formation and calcification of fetal bones and teeth, especially during the third trimester; (20 maintenance of the mother's bones and teeth.

The nonpregnant woman needs 800 milligrams of calcium daily; during pregnancy and lactation the need increases to 1,200.

Good sources of calcium include milk and cheese. The requirement is met by one quart of nonfat or lowfat milk per day.

In addition to the specific nutrients mentioned, you need to have adequate *liquids* in your diet, including water. The pregnant or nonpregnant woman needs four servings of liquids daily. During lactation, the need rises to six servings to help with milk production.

We have included only the main nutrients essential to good health during pregnancy and lactation. An excellent resource for more extensive reading is Phyllis William's *Nourishing Your Unborn Child.*

The "Daily Food Guide" contains protein foods, vegetables, fruits, milk products, and grain products. The following lists of foods, which will help you plan nutritious meals, are adapted from *Nutrition During Pregnancy and lactation.*

Proteins. If you are pregnant or breast feeding, eat four servings of the following:

Animal Protein (complete protein):

As serving is 2 to 3 ounces, cooked and boneless, unless otherwise specified. Beef, poultry, pork, fish, veal, lamb Tuna, salmon, crab, lobster—1/2 cup Shrimp, scallops—6 medium Sausage links—4 Cottage cheese—1/2 cup Cheese—2 ounces Eggs—2 Milk—1 cup

Vegetable Protein (incomplete protein):

A serving is 1 cup cooked, unless otherwise specified. *Note*: These alone will not supply the requirement. See the discussion that follows. Garbanzo, lima, or kidney beans Dried beans or peas Lentils Nuts—1/2 cup Sunflower seeds—1/2 cup Peanut butter—2 tablespoons (without sugar, not hydrogenated) Rice—3/4 cup

Protein is supplied by both animal and vegetable sources. It is either complete or incomplete depending on the number of essential amino acids it contains. Complete protein (milk, cheese, eggs, fish, and meat) contains the essential amino acids in the proper proportions to meet the body's requirements. Incomplete protein (legumes, grains, seeds, nuts) is missing one or more essential amino acids. By serving the incomplete protein with complete protein (cereal and milk, peanut butter and whole wheat bread) or by combining two incomplete proteins (beans and corn), you can have all the essential amino acids. A very good resource on protein is *Diet for a Small Planet* by Frances Moore Lappe. A protein deficiency can cause problems for both the mother and baby.

The chart given on the following page is a guide to help you plan your daily menus.

Milk and *Milk* Products. If you are pregnant, eat 3 to 4 servings of the following. If you are breast feeding, eat 4 to 5 servings.

Milk Products: A serving is 1 cup or 8 ounces, unless otherwise specified.

Cheeses—1 1/2 ounces

Cottage cheese—1 1/3 cups

Milk—whole, nonfat, lowfat, nonfat dry reconstituted, or buttermilk.

Creamed soup—12 ounces or 1 1/2 cups

Ice cream—1 1/2 cups

Ice milk

Milk shake

Pudding

Yogurt

Dry milk—3 to 4 tablespoons

Daily Food Guide

Food Group	*Number Of Servings*		
	Non-pregnant	*Pregnant*	*Breast-feeding*
Protein Group (Animal and Vegetable)	3	4	4
Milk and Milk Products Group	3	4	5
Grain Products Group	3	3	3
Vitamin C Fruits and Vegetables Group	1	1	1
Leafy Green Vegetables Group	2	2	2
Other Yellow Fruits and Vegetables Group	1	1	1

1. Buy only fresh dairy products. Bacteria multiply rapidly when milk is left at room temperature, so refrigeration is essential.
2. Natural cheeses are preferable to processed chesses and spreads which contain many additives. Read the labels.
3. Flavored yogurts contain sugar. Plain yogurt can be flavored with fresh fruit.
4. A quart of milk daily provides excellent protein as well as one-fourth of your daily energy needs. There are many ways to incorporate milk into the diet; for example, dried milk may be added to meat loaf, puddings, soups and sauces.

Grain Products. If you are pregnant or breast feeding, eat three of the following daily.

Whole Grain Products:

Brown rice—1/2 cup

Cereals (hot): oatmeal, rolled wheat, cracked wheat, malted barley—1/2 cup

Cereals (cold): puffed oats, shredded wheat, what flakes, granola—3/4 cup (read label to note amount of sugar and additives)

Cracked and whole wheat bread—1 slice

Wheat germ—1 tablespoon

1. Whole grain products are often more nutritious and provide more fiber than enriched products. It is possible to buy lasagna, spaghetti, noodles, pancake mix, and so on made with whole wheat flour.
2. When you bake use whole wheat or unbleached white flours since they are more nutritious. Use part soy flour when baking for extra nutrition.
3. When baking, use the Cornell Triple Rich Flour Formula. In the bottom of a measuring cup please: 1 tablespoon soy flour, 1 tablespoon dry milk, 1 teaspoon wheat germ. Add flour to make one cup.

Enriched Grain Products:

Bread—1 slice

Hot cereals: cream of wheat of rice—1/2 cup

Cornbread—2-inch square

Crackers—4

Macaroni, spaghetti, noodles—1/2 cup cooked

Muffin, biscuit, or bagel—1

Pancake or waffle—1

Rice—1/2 cup

Corn tortilla—2

Flour tortilla—1

Fruits and Vegetables with Vitamin C. If you are pregnant of breast feeding, eat one of the following daily.

Juices:

Orange or grapefruit – 1/2 cup

Tomato – 1 1/2 cups

Fruit juices enriched with vitamin C – 3/4 cup

Fruits:

Cantaloupe – 1/2

Grapefruit – 1/2

Orange – 1 medium

Strawberries – 3/4 cup

Tangerines – 2 small

Vegetables:

Broccoli – 1 stalk or 1/2 cup

Brussels sprouts – 3-4

Cooked cabbage – 1 1/3 cups

Raw cabbage – 3/4 cup

Green peppers – 1/2 medium

Tomatoes – 2 medium

1. Unless enriched with Vitamin C, canned fruits and juices are lower in Vitamin C content than fresh of frozen.
2. Ascorbic acid is extremely perishable. Exposure to bright light, air, prolonged cooking, preparation in blenders, or soaking in water destroys it.

Leafy Green Vegetables with Vitamin A, Folic acid, and Iron. Choose two of these each day if you are pregnant or breast feeding.

Leafy Green Vegetables: A serving is 1 cup raw or 3/4 cup cooked.

Asparagus

Broccoli

Brussels sprouts Cabbage

Dark leafy lettuce (endive

Greens (beet, collard, kale, spinach, swiss chard, turnip, scallions)

Yellow Fruits and Vegetables with Vitamin A. Choose one of these each day if you are pregnant or breast feeding.

Yellow Fruits: A serving is 1/2 cup unless otherwise specified.

Apricot – 1

Nectarines – 2

Peach – 1

Prunes – 4

Apple – 1

Banana – 1

Berries

Yellow Vegetables: A serving is 1/2 cup unless otherwise specified.

Artichoke

Bean sprouts

Beets

Carrots

Cauliflower

Celery

Corn

Dates – 5
Figs – 2
Grapes
Pear – 1
Pineapple
Plums – 2
Raisins
Watermelon

Cucumber
Eggplant
Beans – green or waxed
Lettuce
Mushrooms
Onions
Peas
Potatoes
Squash
Yams

Consider These Suggestions

1. Generally speaking, fresh is the best, frozen the second, and canned the least nutritious way to buy fruits and vegetables. When buying canned fruits, avoid those packed in syrups, choosing natural juices when available. Look in the diet foods section of your store for fruits packed in water or natural juice. Some major companies now produce lightly sweetened fruits. Be sure to read the label for other additives.
2. Eat raw vegetables or cook minimally, just untill done.
3. Store foods in airtight containers. Wash vegetables just before cooking and avoid long exposure to air. Remember that most vitamins are near the skin so scrub lightly and pare only if necessary. After paring or slicing, cook immediately. Care in preparing vegetables will maximize the nutritional content.
4. Steaming is a preferable way to cook vegetables, and a perforated steamer is an excellent investment. Frying foods increases calories but not nutrition.
5. Another good investment is *The Joy of Cooking*, which describes how to purchase, store, prepare, and serve all kinds of vegetables.

A Few Other Comments about Food

Sugar. Sugar is fifty calories per tablespoon. It contains no vitamins, minerals, or protein. It is a known factor in tooth decay, obesity, and heart disease, yet it is present in most processed foods—even those that don't taste sweet. It should have a minimal part in your diet. Sweetness can be supplied by fresh fruits and unsweetened juices. Check your area for classes in sugarless cooking methods.

When your baby begins to eat foods, you might want to look at Vicki Lansky's *The Taming of the C.A.N.D.Y. Monster (Continuously Advertised Nutritionally Deficient Yummies).*

Additives. "The food industry puts more than 1 billion pounds of chemicals per year into the processed foods you and I eat. This averages out to about five pounds per person annually."

Not all additives have been proven safe. The more fresh, unprocessed foods you eat, the better.

Labels. Read labels. The ingredients are listed in the order of their prevalence in the product: the ingredient listed first is found in the greatest quantity, and so on.

An excellent investment is *The Supermarket handbook* by Nikki and David Goldbeck.

Feeding Your Baby

Although it is early to be thinking about your baby's diet, here are some points to consider now and again later.

To help prevent allergic reactions, many pediatricians recommend waiting six months before introducing solid foods. During the second six months of your baby's life, slowly introduce solids and continue to breast feed or formula feed your baby. It is often suggested that you delay switching to cow's milk until the child is one year old, especially if your family has a history of allergies.

When you do introduce solids, you will choose between the commercially prepared and home prepared foods. if you purchase the former, be sure to read the labels. Sugar, salt, tapioca, and other additives and unnecessary additions to baby food. There are now many commercially made baby foods that do not have additives and are high in vitamins and minerals.

You may want to make some of all of your own baby food. If so, make sure that you use fresh, quality produce and meats. Cook produce minimally so you retain most of the vitamins and minerals. Do not add sugar or salt. Make sure your utensils and pots are absolutely clean.

Prepare in quantity whenever possible. For instance, cook a two- pound bag of carrots and then grind or puree them. You can fill an ice tray with the carrot mixture. When frozen, put the carrot cubes in a plastic freezer bag and store in the freezer until you need them. Warm them in a baby food dish or in a pyrex dish in boiling water.

28

The Later Trimester

This chapter includes emotional changes and sexuality during the third trimester, warning signs during pregnancy, preparation for childbirth, breast feeding, and buying wisely for your baby.

Changes

The final three months of pregnancy, known as the third trimester, mark a shift toward active preparation for the birth of the baby. Couples take childbirth preparation classes, decorate the nursery, and choose names for their babies. They begin to think of themselves less as a pregnant couple and more as parents with new responsibilities.

The Mother's Emotional Reactions

The last trimester is usually the time of most physical discomfort. You will probably be very ready for the baby to be born, even though you are nostalgic about the end of this special time in your life. The heightened sensitivity and mood swings you have earlier in pregnancy continue.

Fears about childbirth are common. You are about to experience something totally new, and to fear the unknown is natural. You may wonder whether you can cope with labor and delivery, how you will act, whether there will be pain, and about the health of your baby.

Women are often engrossed in conversations about children and dreams of their babies. At the time of birth, the child you had imagined will have to be emotionally replaced with the real child. Sometimes it can be an adjustment, especially if a child of the opposite sex was expected or the baby's physical appearance is very different than imagined.

Because of your physical appearance—an enlarged abdomen, large breasts, clumsiness, and so on—your body image may change. You may doubt your physical attractiveness, especially to your mate. On the other hand, some women feel beautiful throughout pregnancy.

The Father's Emotional Reactions

The father's emotions also become directed toward the reality of the baby and the end of pregnancy. Concerns over the safety of the baby and mother during labor and delivery are common. Your thoughts are often filled with questions about fatherhood. "What kind of father will I be?" "Will I be able to provide enough financial security?" It is a time of increased awareness of the meaning of family.

In addition to these concerns, you are also involved in those of the mother and in her increased emotional sensitivity. Now is an important time to offer reassurance that her changing shape is desirable and that together you can cope with labor, delivery, and parenthood.

Very crucial to this time in pregnancy is open communication or discussion of feelings and concerns between father and mother. Childbirth education classes are another source of reassurance to a couple. The information from class can decrease fears, increase knowledge, and provide positive tools to use in labor and delivery. Also, the social experience with other couples is invaluable; usually you learn that you are all having many of the same emotions and concerns.

Sexual Relations

How couples feel about sex during the last three months of pregnancy can vary greatly. Some couples feel an interest in lovemaking and continue to have intercourse through these last months. They are able to overcome the obstacles of a larger, cumbersome uterus and the mother's awkward movements by experimenting with new positions and new forms of physical closeness. Positions may include facing each other while side-lying, rear entry, woman superior, and so on. Other couples experience a decline in sexual interest or may decide to limit or restrict intercourse during the last months. Sometimes physicians counsel against intercourse or lovemaking that results in maternal orgasm, perhaps because of vaginal bleeding, ruptured membranes, a deeply engaged presenting part, incompetent cervix, or pain during intercourse.

Women can have mixed feelings about their bodies. To some women, their enlarged, redefined bodies—swollen breasts, large abdomen, awkward movements, and increased vaginal secretions—are disturbing. They may feel embarrassed or dislike their bodies, which can influence how they feel about relations with their mate. other women seem to blossom and take real delight in their womanliness. They may have a continued or even increased sexual desire.

Men can have equally varied feelings regarding their mate's changing body and the impending delivery of their baby. Some men take great interest in the enlarging body and fetal movements. The woman may take on special qualities to the man, and her fertility adds a special quality to their lovemaking. New positions, as well as new forms of sexual behavior, may appeal to some men and not to others. Some men feel uncomfortable with the physical appearance of their mate. They may be concerned about injuring the baby during intercourse or initiating labor.

Following are some of the physical facts regarding intercourse during the third trimester:

1. Before your baby's birth, there is little risk of infection unless the membranes are ruptured and bacteria from the vagina can enter the amniotic sac.
2. Masters and Johnson concluded from a study on pregnant women that orgasm can initiate labor if the mother is near term and conditions for labor are ripe.
3. Toward the end of pregnancy, the increased size of the woman's abdomen may necessitate a change in position. Excessive pressure should not be put on the pregnant uterus. When the baby's head drops lower in the pelvis, an erect penis may be uncomfortable for the woman, but it is not likely that the penis can rupture the membranes. Questions about sexual relations as they pertain to your own medical condition can be discussed with your physician.

Whether the couple continues to have intercourse or whether there is a decline in sexual activity, it is important that the lines of communication be kept open. Being frank and honest in your discussions about how you feel can be beneficial to you as a couple. The way you feel is not wrong; feelings are legitimate. Many couples increasingly need affection, closeness, tenderness, kissing, and touching. These are other ways of expressing love and can make the last months of pregnancy a time of closeness—emotionally and physically. An excellent resource ia *Making Love During Pregnancy* by Bing and Colman.

Warning Signs During Pregnancy

Call your doctor if any of these occur:

1. Pain or burning when you urinate, or a decrease in the amount of urine
2. Vaginal bleeding or spotting
3. Persistent headache
4. Swelling or puffiness (retention of fluid) in hands, feet, face
5. Sharp abdominal pain or severe cramping. Nausea or queasy feeling in stomach
6. Rupture or leakage of amniotic fluid
7. Fever of 100 degrees or higher
8. Dizziness
9. Blurred vision
10. Any illness you have

Toxemia

Toxemia is a condition of pregnancy with several different symptoms, including

- Hypertension—the mother's blood pressure rises.
- Edema—fluid accumulates in the mother's body, especially in her hands and face.
- Proteinuria—protein or albumin is present in the mother's urine.

These symptoms are easily identifiable and should be checked at each prenatal visit.

Mild toxemia is termed pre-eclampsia. If the mother's blood pressure increases, she has protein in the urine, and/or edema, she is said to have pre-eclampsia. She may have had a sudden weight gain, headaches, blurred vision, nausea, vomiting, a decrease in the amount of urine, and emotional tension. When the condition becomes more severe it is called eclampsia.

The causes of toxemia are not completely understood. It occurs most often in women younger than 20 or older than 30 having their first babies, in multiple pregnancies, in women with more than five pregnancies, and in nonwhites.

Treatment for toxemia is very important, and women should watch for symptoms between prenatal visits. Treatment usually includes bed rest of one's left side with the feet elevated. A diet with adequate protein is encouraged. Excessive salt should be avoided, but the elimination of all salt is discouraged. Toxemia can often be controlled with these measures, but delivery is the only way to eliminate the disease.

Preparation for Childbirth

Everyone who comes to the experience of childbirth is prepared. The crux of the matter is whether the preparation is positive and realistic or negative and inaccurate.

Unfortunately, many of us approach childbirth with negative expectations. For centuries most cultures have held that pain is inevitable during childbirth. Rarely have television shows, books, or movies expounded on the thrill and excitement of childbirth; rather, they dwell on the pain, which seldom is portrayed as controllable. Your culture has influenced your mental attitude toward childbirth and will influence how your perceive you labor contractions. stories told to you by your mother, friends, and relatives about their childbirths or your own observations and previous experience can also affect how you feel about childbirth, and consequently, how you will react to your labor and delivery.

During the third trimester, many expectant couples find themselves anticipating the impending childbirth experience with some apprehension. The purpose of childbirth education is to prepare couples to deal positively with the birth experience. They are educated about the process of labor and delivery, they are taught techniques to deal with the mother's discomfort and pain, and they are informed about the variations that can occur. Most couples begin childbirth preparation during their third trimester.

Lamaze

Lamaze is one method of childbirth preparation. It is a "man-made", not a "natural", method of dealing with labor contractions, and it prepares you emotionally, intellectually, and physically for childbirth. Its primary goal is to have a healthy mother deliver a healthy baby. It offers you psychological techniques, or tools, you can use during your labor to make it a more shared, enjoyable, and meaningful experience. Lamaze techniques have been proven to be beneficial in decreasing the mother's perception of pain during labor and delivery.

The basis of Lamaze originated in Russia where women were conditioned or trained to respond to their contractions with relaxation. In the 1950s, Fernand Lamaze, a Frenchman, adapted the Russian techniques and introduced his method of prepared childbirth. The conditioned, or automatic, response is still the basis, but Lamaze added special breathing techniques to the Russian method. In the United States the method has been expanded to include fathers in a coaching role, allowing couples to share actively in the birth of their child. Today, Lamaze is a very popular method to control the pain of labor.

Causes of Pain During Childbirth

During childbirth the woman must deal with two different sources of pain—one during labor; the other during delivery. The anatomy of childbirth is thoroughly discussed later, but briefly the following is what occurs:

Your baby is now securely inside a muscle called the uterus of womb, which looks like an upside-down pear with a small opening at the bottom. This lower portion of the uterus is your cervix. During labor the cervix has to open enough for your baby to pass through; it has to change from a very small opening to one about four inches across. This miraculous event occurs because the muscle fibers of your uterus are capable of contracting, or getting shorter, and then relaxing, or lengthening. These are the labor contractions about which you've probably heard. Contractions push the baby's head against the cervix, causing it to open. Pain during labor is primarily caused by the opening of your cervix. During the pushing or delivery stage, however, pain is mostly caused by the stretching and pressure which occur as the baby moves down the birth canal (or vagina).

Perception of Pain During Childbirth

Sensations (stimuli) during labor and delivery travel through nerve fibers up the spinal cord to the brain, which interprets them. You respond behavioraly depending on your interpretation. Unprepared women respond by tensing, screaming, and becoming frightened. Prepared women respond by using breathing and relaxation techniques.

How your brain perceives or interprets labor contractions or how much discomfort you actually feel depends on a number of factors:

1. *Fear:* How anxious or frightened are you about your labor and delivery? Your level of anxiety plays a large part in determining how you will interpret and respond to uterine contractions. Anxiety sets up a negative cycle, called the fear-tension-pain cycle, which is often seen in untrained laboring women. Their fear makes them become tense, which increases the pain, which in turn makes them more frightened, and the cycle repeats.
2. *Physical factors:* Are you healthy and well rested when you go into labor? How long since you last ate? How close together and strong are your contractions? How long have you been in labor?

3. *Emotional factors*: Are you highly motivated to use Lamaze techniques? Is your labor coach supportive? Do you feel comfortable where you're laboring and with the birth attendants caring for you?
4. *Focus of attention:* Are you attending to the intensity of the contractions or is your focus of attention elsewhere? Are you actively using the techniques taught in childbirth education classes?

Increasing Your Pain Threshold

Richard Stevens, a neurophysiologist, has presented research on psychological strategies, or techniques, which enable people to tolerate more pain, or increase their pain threshold.

1. *Active relaxation:* relaxing the muscles in your body except the uterus.
2. *Cognitive control*: using mind to help deal with pain.
   a. *Disassociation:* concentrating on a nonpainful aspect of the stimulus, or contraction.
   b. *Focusing attention:* actively involving your mind with techniques, such as breathing patterns, instead of thinking about your contractions.
3. *Rehearsal:* becoming educated to reduce your fear of the unknown.
4. *Hawthorne effect:* someone important to the laboring mother giving her attention, namely, the coach, the staff, and the physician.

Using Psychological Strategies

Lamaze can help you use these psychological strategies to raise your pain threshold in the following ways.

1. *Active relaxation:* You will be trained to actively or consciously relax during labor contractions, and your coach will be trained to help you. Instead of reacting to a contraction with tension, you will be taught to relax your muscles.
2. *Disassociation:* In Lamaze we speak about labor contractions not labor pains. You will learn to think of a contraction as the mechanism causing your cervix to open so your baby can be born.
3. *Focusing attention:* Your mind will be occupied with the Lamaze techniques—breathing patterns, relaxation, massage, and focusing your eyes on an object in the room. For example, concentrating on the discomfort of a headache increases the pain, whereas engaging your mind elsewhere decreases your awareness of the

headache. In the same manner, focusing your attention on Lamaze techniques will keep your mind so occupied that you will be less aware of the uterine contractions.

4. *Cognitive rehearsal:* One of the purposes of Lamaze classes and this book is to teach you about the childbirth process.

   This knowledge will enable you to mentally and physically rehearse what will occur during labor, eliminating many of the fears and anxieties you may have from misinformation or lack of information.

5. *Hawthorne effect:* Having a labor coach who practices with you before labor and is with you throughout labor and delivery insures that you have help and attention. Your coach should be someone to whom you are close emotionally. A study on the effect of a husband or coach on the perception of pain determined that practical help was more effective than only moral support. Lamaze teaches your coach specific ways to assist you. Another positive influence is the time your nurse and doctor spend with you, helping with techniques or keeping you informed about your labor.

In summary, you can psychologically or physiologically manage the pain of childbirth. Your mind interprets sensations from your body. You can block your awareness of the sensations coming from the uterine contractions by occupying your mind with the psychological strategies just listed. You can also block or decrease painful stimuli by using physical means, such as light massage (effleurage), on the surface of your body.

Your goal is to make the Lamaze techniques become automatic responses to uterine contractions. Instead of becoming tense and frightened you will automatically relax and use special breathing patterns. This change in behavior occurs through practice. Just as riding a bicycle becomes automatic after practice, so will your Lamaze techniques.

It is important for both you and your coach to rehearse your labor roles daily. You need to learn to respond to your coach's touch, voice, and presence. At the same time, the coach learns how to help your relax and what techniques work best for you. You will become a labor team. Stevens reports that the more time you practice your techniques, the more effective they become. In addition to the technical reasons, the time you devote to practice illustrates your emotional support for each other in the preparation for the birth of your child.

During your third trimester you will need to make some decisions regarding the care of your baby, for example, the method of feeding and what clothes and equipment to purchase. Here are a few facts that you may want to consider.

Breast Feeding

Until modern times and in less industrialized and affluent societies, breast feeding has been the accepted method of feeding babies. With affluence came the prestige of being able to afford to bottle feed babies. Breast feeding also diminished in popularity as a woman's breasts began to be seen as more of a sex symbol.

However, in recent years there has been a renewed interest in breast feeding, especially among couples taking childbirth preparation classes. If you haven't already, you should begin now to decide how you will feed your baby. This decision deserves consideration from both parents. After you have an intellectual understanding of breast feeding, sit down and discuss how each of you feels about it emotionally.

Benefits

1. *Nutrition:* Breast milk is perfectly suited to an infant, and it is more easily digested than cow's milk. Breast-fed babies usually don't require additional sources of nutrition until 4 to 6 months of age.

   Immunities: Immunities are passed to the baby through colostrum, the substance produced by the breast during pregnancy. The baby drinks colostrum until the mother's milk comes in.

3. *Convenience:* Breast milk is always ready, the right temperature, and easily transported on trips.
4. *Emotional gratification:* Breast feeding fosters a close physical and emotional relationship between a mother and her nursing baby. It is gratifying to be able to supply your baby with the nourishment she needs.
5. *Economics:* Breast feeding requires that the mother consume an extra five hundred calories per day. This food and perhaps supplemental vitamins are your only extra expenses. Bottle feeding can be an obvious addition to the family food bill.
6. *Time:* No preparations are necessary for breast feeding other than a nutritious diet and rest when you're trying to establish your milk supply those first few weeks. You need the rest to recover from childbirth anyway. Preparing bottles and formula takes time, which would be more fun to spend with your baby. There's also no heating bottles at 2:00A.M. while your baby cries, waiting to be fed.
7. *Allergies:* Breast-fed babies are less likely to develop allergies to milk. The sooner cow's milk and solids are introduced, the more likely a child is to develop an allergic reaction.

8. *Obesity:* Breast-fed babies are usually not overfed. If the baby has frequent wet diapers you can assume he is getting enough to eat. The baby simply nurses until satisfied. Bottle-fed babies are sometimes encouraged to finish the bottle, and consequently, are overfed. Recent studies are beginning to show that the extra fat cells we acquire as babies stay with us and contribute to weight problems later on.

9. *Dental development:* The sucking action at the breast fosters good jaw and facial muscle development.

10. *Bowel movements:* The stools of a breast-fed baby are loose and the odor is mild. Constipation is rarely a problem.

Breast Function

There are two main things you need to understand about your milk supply. First, milk is produced as a result of a hormone called *prolactin* and the sucking of your baby. How much the baby nurses determines how much milk the breast produces. It stands to reason, then, that a newborn will want to eat frequently to build up your milk supply. Second, when your baby begins to nurse, the sucking stimulates your pituitary gland to release a hormone called *oxytocin*. This reaction causes the milk to be let down from the milk ducts so the baby can get it. Your letdown reflex is strongly affected by emotions. If you are tense, worried, or in some way emotionally upset, you will not relax enough for the milk to let down. Then you end up with a frustrated mother and a hungry baby. This problem is bound to occur sometime to any nursing mother, so try to remedy the situation with some conscious relaxation, a hot shower, a little beer or wine, imagining the milk letting down, and removing the source of anxiety, if possible.

Preparing the Nipples

The value of this preparation during pregnancy seems to lend itself to controversy. Many women never have sore nipples from breast feeding, but others do. It is generally believed that fair-complexioned people are more susceptible. Many women believe it was beneficial for them to have done some or all of the following during the last few weeks of pregnancy to toughen their nipples.

1. Pull the nipples out slightly and roll them between thumb and finger. This exercise will make the nipple more erect and easier for your baby to grasp.

2. Discontinue using soap on your nipples because it tends to dry the skin, making them more susceptible to cracking.

3. Rub the nipples with a terry towel and expose them to the air and your clothing, by occasionally not wearing a bra.

4. Hand express colostrum. It is believed by some to open the milk ducts and possibly decrease engorgement.

Beginning to Breast Feed

First, you need to realize that it takes to establish a milk supply and time for you and the baby to learn to breast feed. Some babies nurse right away and others lick the nipple and seem initially disinterested. They need time to learn. Also, it is easier for some mothers than it is for others.

When should you start? Some women are comfortable nursing in the delivery room. Others prefer to wait until they get to recovery and can adjust their position more easily. Be sure to ask for help if you need it. The nurse can show you how to get the nipple in the baby's mouth and how to position yourself for comfort. No one expects you to know how to nurse if you've never done it before.

At first your baby will be getting colostrum, not milk. This substance is full of protein and immunities and is usually all your baby needs those first few days. Your milk will come in about 2 to 4 days after birth. Most women's breasts become engorged when their milk comes in; the breasts become sore and swollen because of the inelasticity of the milk ducts. This condition usually subsides as soon as the milk supply adjusts and the milk ducts become more elastic. Sometimes heat (a hot bath) or hand expressing some milk will relieve some of the soreness.

Nurse your baby as frequently as he seems hungry. If your hospital allows rooming-in, take advantage of it so your baby will be with you when he gets hungry. Start right away to drink plenty of fluids. It takes about 2 to 3 quarts of fluids a day for you to produce milk and maintain you own body's hydration.

Once you get home be sure to get plenty of rest and drink something each time you nurse. Ignore the housework temporarily and take advantage of relatives' or friends' offers to help with a meal or the house.

It might take four to six weeks before your milk supply is established and you and the baby are really comfortable nursing. During this time it is very important for you to have someone you can call on to answer your questions. This person might be a friend who has breast-fed, your Lamaze instructor, or a member of Laleche League, an organization of nursing mothers available to help you. Select a doctor for your baby who supports breast feeding and can answer your questions.

Persevere. Soon you and the baby will be a happy breast feeding team.

If you're beginning to feel tied down, remember how easily your baby can go out with you. Short outings will be less tiring. You might have a friend baby-sit while you go out for an hour after feeding the baby.

Obstacles to Breast Feeding

Some women develop sore nipples when they begin to breast feed. Usually the discomfort is noticed most when the infant first starts to suck. Some of the following might help:

- Expose the nipple to air and sun (don't get burned).
- Use pure hydrous lanolin on the nipples after each feeding to keep them supple. (It can be purchased at a pharmacy). Lanolin does not have to be wiped off before your baby nurses the next time.
- Don't wait so long between feedings that your breasts become full and the baby can't grasp the nipple easily.
- Change nursing positions for each feeding.
- Avoid nursing bras or nursing pads with plastic liners; they don't allow air to get to your nipples.

Mastitis, or a breast infection, sometimes occurs. Completely emptying your breasts of milk at each feeding allows for good drainage and usually insures against mastitis, but not always. If you notice a red spot on your breast of have a fever and feel like you're getting the flu, call your doctor immediately. If you treat an infection in the beginning, it usually does not become bothersome. The usual treatment includes (1) moist heat on the area of infection, (2) antibiotics, (3) rest, and (4) continued nursing on the affected breast (since the usual cause of the infection is incomplete emptying of the milk).

As a preventive measure, be sure to alternate the side on which you begin nursing. Nursing in different positions (sitting up, lying down) will also help to insure that the baby completely empties the milk ducts.

The attitudes of your friends and relatives who are negative about breast feeding can be difficult to deal with when you're first starting to nurse. The first time the baby fusses after you've fed him and your friend suggests you don't have enough milk, you wonder just a little if it's true.

Worrying about it can affect your milk supply, so be confident and ask your friend not to interfere.

Finally, life can be miserable if you feed your baby be the clock. Your baby is the best judge of when he's hungry. On the other hand, don't get into the routine of feeding him every hour round the clock, you'll both be exhausted.

Is it worth it? Ask any breast-feeding mother who's past the initial adjustment and she'll say yes. The close relationship with the baby and the confidence in being able to nurture your child are very gratifying.

Fathers Can Help

First and foremost, fathers can help by offering their encouragement and emotional support. Your mate needs to know that you want her to succeed and are willing to help her. You can help by insisting that she rest when the baby rests and reminding her to drink plenty of fluids. You can help initially by bringing her the baby at night, straightening the house, and fixing some of the meals. Be flexible. Your dinner may be late occasionally; babies always seem to eat right at the dinner hour.

Some fathers think that because they don't actually feed the baby they aren't needed. Nothing could be more incorrect. The baby needs your love just as much as the mother's. Enjoy your baby, learn to diaper and care for him, and help him get to know you. Relax and be confidant that your baby is being well nourished in a very natural way.

Deciding to Bottle Feed

If you decide that bottle feeding is more suitable for you and your baby, have confidence in your decision and enjoy this experience with your baby. You can develop the same nurturing, close relationship as long as you hold and cuddle your baby while you feed him. *Please* don't prop the bottle.

Follow the advice of your baby's doctor about formulas and bottles. You can feed the baby on demand and let him eat as much as he wants; he might not need the last two ounces in the bottle. A real benefit of bottle feeding is that the father can enjoy feeding the baby too.

Buying for Your Baby

You are about to embark on what is an expensive venture—the raising of a child. By careful planning before you shop, however, you can make or buy equipment, clothing, and toys of good quality and still be economical. One source calculates that raising one child is 15 to 17 per cent of the yearly family income, so careful shopping is important.

Make a list of the things you will need before you go shopping. Find out what is considered good quality for each item and what the safety requirements are. Your local Consumer Safety Commission office has free information, or you can write to the Washington office: U.S. Consumer Products Safety Commission, Washington, D.C. 21207. another source of information is *Consumers Union Guide to Buying for Babies, published by Consumer Reports*. This book rates many baby articles: cribs, diapers, sleepers, carriages, bike seats, gates, vaporizers, pins, pacifiers, and so on.

The following discussion considers some major pieces of equipment.

Car Seat. A car seat is an important investment, and the purchase of a safe one should be high on your list of priorities. You should have one in which to bring your baby home from the hospital.

Two sources to consult are (1) *Consumer Reports magazine,* June 1977 (or the latest article); and (2) "Don't Risk Your Child's Life" (1976), published by Physicians for Automotive Safety, 50 Union Avenue, Irvington, New Jersey 07111. Keep in mind that some companies make one car seat only for babies and a different model for an older child. Other companies make models that can be used for both ages. Follow the manufacturer's suggestions for installation to maximize safety.

Cribs and Highchairs. A safe crib and highchair are two other important, costly investments. To be sure that you understand the safety features of each, consult your local Consumer Safety Commission office, write to the national office requesting their pamphlets, or read *Consumer's Guide.* Most new products meet these requirements, but if you plan to refurbish an antique or accept a hand-me-down, do yourself and your baby a favor and find out how to make it safe.

Baby Carrier. Many new mothers and fathers find these a wonderful invention for getting out or for dealing with a fussy baby. The Snugli is a well-made corduroy or seersucker infant carrier, which allows you to carry the baby on your chest or back and leaves your arms free. Many stores carry them, they can sometimes be bought used or borrowed from friends; or you can write to Snugli Cottage Industries, Route 7, Box 685A, Evergreen, Colorado 80439. Check with a children's store about other types of baby carriers or packs.

Toys. For information on toy safety write to Toys, Washington, D.C. 20207; the toll-free number is (800) 638–2666. For an exhaustive description of age-appropriate, good-quality toys, books, and music, consult the appendix on *How To Parent* by Fitzhugh Dobson.

Diapers. Diapers are a major investment whether you buy cloth or disposable diapers or use a diaper service. Many parents use a combination of all three. Consult *Consumer's Guide* for information on each type of diaper.

A diaper service supplies you with a specific number of diapers in the size you request (ask for the newborn size initially). All you do is rinse the diapers; the company picks up soiled diapers and delivers clean ones. If your baby has very sensitive skin, this may be your best option. Call companies in your areas to compare prices and service.

For cloth diapers, an initial investment is required in the purchase of five or six dozen diapers, after which there are maintenance costs—hot water, soap, dryer, and so on. You of course, are responsible for rinsing, washing, drying, and folding diapers. Care must be taken to rinse the diapers thoroughly when laundering to avoid irritating the baby's sensitive skin.

Cloth diapers come in different sizes, weights, and quality. Invest in good diapers and a size that your child won't outgrow, you can always fold them smaller for a newborn. After your baby is through with the diapers, you can use them for your next child, and later you will have a large supply of dustcloths.

Disposable diapers are convenient but can be expensive and of questionable value environmentally. Also they irritate some babies' skin. They come in different sizes, depending on your baby's age and weight, and have different absorbencies, depending on the manufacturer and whether they are for the day or night. They vary considerably in quality and price.

Many parents choose to use a combination of the above. Ask for diaper service as a gift, or treat yourself during the immediate postpartum period. Buy your own diapers and use them most of the time. Use disposable diapers when you go out, or as a treat occasionally. Watch for sales.

Infants' Wear. A basic layette for a baby includes diapers, six to ten pairs of rubber pants, and a few crib sheets. A summer baby will probably do well in undershirts and a sun-shielding hat or bonnet. A few sunsuits are nice but not necessary. A winter infant requires more clothing: undershirts and six to twelve uncomplicated, front-opening stretch suits (one-piece stretch terry outfits). It's hard to have too many of these. They are so useful that the baby can wear them in the day and sleep in them at night; or you can invest in a few nightgowns (long gowns with string closing at the bottom) and a few heavier blanket sleepers.

Blankets are necessary. Lightweight ones are good for summer, but in the winter you'll also need some heavier ones. Square blankets are best. Consider making your own out of lightweight, 45-inch wide, flame-resistant flannel.

Be cautious about the three-month size. The garment may look big to you while you are pregnant, but babies are notorious for rapidly out-growing those little sizes. Your baby will do nicely with one special out-fit. Somehow those fancy little dresses and suits don't get used very much.

Even if you plan to use disposables or diaper service, buy a dozen diapers for your own use. They are drool pads, burp pads, changing pads, and have all kinds of other uses.

Be sure to follow the laundering directions on the labels of your baby's clothing to maintain their flame-resistant quality.

Things To Do Before Your Baby's Birthday

Things for the baby:

– 1. Make early arrangements for diaper service if you plan to use one, or watch newspapers for sales on disposable diapers.

– 2. Watch newspapers for sales on baby clothes and cloth diapers.

– 3. Launder and put away baby clothes.

– 4. If you plan to bottle feed, have formula and necessary equipment your doctor recommends on hand.

– 5. Have on hand nursery items, such as powder, soap, oil, cornstarch, etc. Discuss with your doctor what products he prefers. Some doctors are particular about what they want you to use.

– 6. If breast feeding, read a book on nursing and take it with you to the hospital.

– 7. Buy or borrow a car seat for an infant, and plan to use it from the very beginning. Try it in your car to make sure that it fits the car's seat belts.

Things for the parents:

– 1. Cook or bake several casseroles and freeze them. Solicit offers of meals from your friends.

– 2. Plan a week of menus, and stock your freezer and pantry for these meals. Fresh fruit, vegetables, and dairy products can be bought later.

– 3. Start looking for baby-sitter possibilities. An exchange of baby-sitting with some members of your childbirth preparation class is a good possibility.

– 4. Buy, address, and stamp birth announcements. You can fill in the vital statistics in the hospital. If you're planning to design on original birth announcement, have some ideas ready and a printer or copying place in mind.

– 5. Buy presents and cards for the birthdays and other occasions that occur around your due date.

– 6. Buy sanitary pads for the first weeks at home.

– 7. If you are breast feeding, buy nursing bras, two front-opening nightgowns, and nursing pads. You can make your own pads from soft, absorbent material or use handerchiefs.

– 8. Do not prematurely pack away your maternity clothes. These or other loose-fitting clothing will be more comfortable for the first few weeks.

– 9. Have plenty of film on hand.

– 10. Pack your suitcase for the hospital.

Include hare any other things you would like to accomplish before your baby is born.

Choosing A Doctor for Your Baby

The decision about who will care for your baby (whether a pediatrician or a family practitioner) is an important one. It should be made during your third trimester, long before your due date.

Try to think of yourself as a health consumer. You will want the best possible care for your new baby. Sometimes it is hard for those without children to really know what's important. One thing you can do is talk to friends who already have children and find out their priorities. Also, make a list of your concerns and needs. Then interview some doctors. A face-to-face meeting is usually more productive than a phone call. Ask the doctor how she sees her role as provider of health care for your baby. Go over your list of questions and concerns. Finally, evaluate your feelings about the doctor. Can you communicate? Is she reassuring? Try to think of her as more than just a baby doctor. Do you think you will feel comfortable discussing problems with her? Often the doctor cares for the parents as much as she cares for the baby during the first year.

In the space below, make a list of questions for discussion with prospective pediatricians or family practitioners. These topics may stimulate some questions: feeding theories, what to do in an emergency, availability by phone, knowledge and screening of developmental growth, knowledge and interest in helping parents deal with behaviour problems, fees, and opinion regarding circumcision.

29

Comfort and Exercise

This chapter includes information to help you look and feel better during your pregnancy and to help you prepare for labor and delivery. Posture, comfort positions, prenatal exercises, and the pelvic floor are discussed.

Posture

Good posture maintained throughout your pregnancy and for the rest of your life will help you feel more energetic and more comfortable. Many of the common aches and pains associated with pregnancy can be prevented or alleviated if you stand and sit properly. By aligning your body correctly, you relieve stress on muscles, joints, and ligaments, and the uterus will maintain its proper position in the pelvic cavity.

Standing

Imagine that a string is attached to the crown of your head and is pulling you up, trying to make you stand straight.

1. You will find that your chin should be tucked in just a little, to align your head with your body. Many people walk around as if they are in a big hurry, with their heads preceding their bodies.

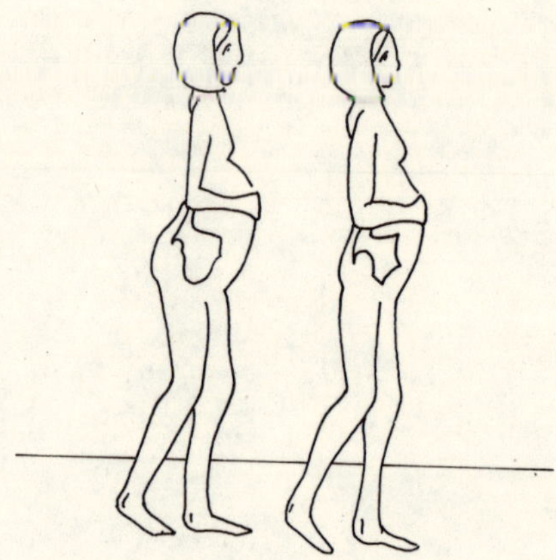

Incorrect Posture – Pelvis tilted forward – Back is swayed
Correct Posture – Pelvis tilted backward – Back is straight

2. Your shoulders should be pulled back slightly. Rounded shoulders are a common postural defect.

3. Your pelvis should be tilted backward so your low back is straight, not swayed. To get your pelvis back, you need to tuck in your but tocks and pull in your stomach.

4. Your knees should be slightly flexed, or bent, and your feet should be pointed forward.

5. Most of your weight is on the outer borders of your feet.

Check your posture by leaning against a wall with your feet about five inches away. Tilt your pelvis backward so that your entire back is touching the wall. Now step away from the wall and see if you can maintain this posture while you walk. Do not walk stiffly, but simply make an effort to hold in your stomach and tuck in your buttocks. An occasional glance into the mirror can help you determine if your back is straight or swayed.

Poor posture stretches and weakens abdominal muscles while tightening back muscles, resulting in increased stress on joints, ligaments, and muscles. Backache is often the result of poor posture. If you need to stand for prolonged periods at work or perhaps waiting in line, you can prevent your pelvis from tipping forward by placing one foot on a step or stool. This position automatically tilts the pelvis back and reduces the sway in your back. Avoid wearing high-heeled shoes, as they throw your weight forward, and to compensate, you arch your back.

To prevent pooling of blood in your legs while standing, shift your weight from one foot to the other or rock back and forth on your heels and toes. This exercise helps the leg muscles force the blood up out of your legs. Excessive pooling of blood in your legs results in varicose veins and can reduce your blood pressure, causing a subsequent feeling of faintness or dizziness. Always sit down if you start to feel light-headed.

Sitting

Because many of us sit for prolonged periods of time at work or school, it is important to sit correctly. While sitting, elevate your legs when possible and get up as often as you can to stretch and walk around.

1. If you are sitting in an upright chair, tilt your pelvis back, moving your bottom slightly forward away from the back of the chair seat. Do not slump in your chair.

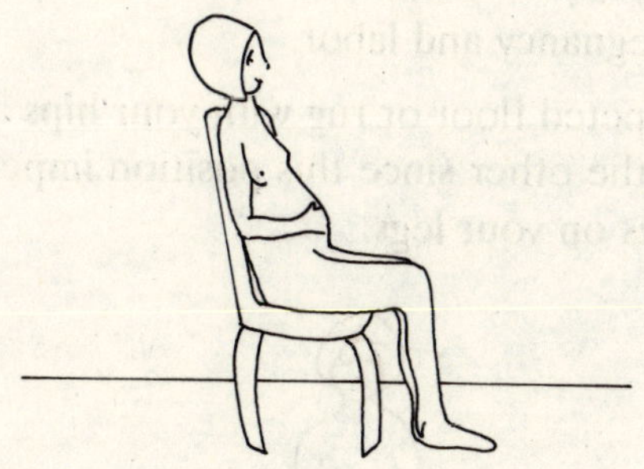

Comfort Sitting Posture

2. If you are leaning forward in a chair, as in typing or writing, sit with your buttocks against the back of the chair, lean your body forward, and keep your back straight, not swayed. In other words, don't throw your shoulders back in order to sit up straight as this posture only increases the curve in your lower back.

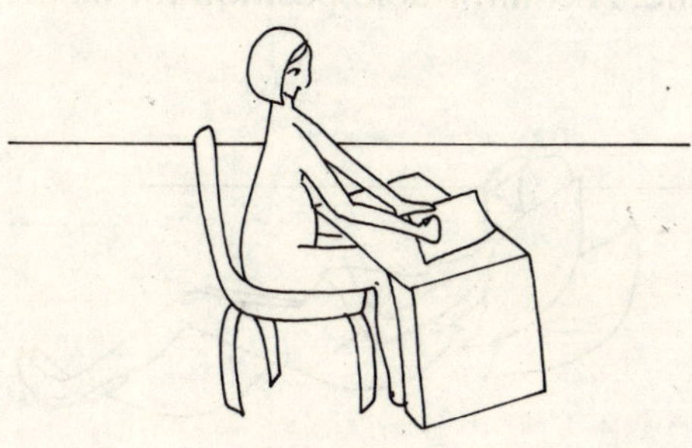

Correct Sitting Posture

Comfort Positions

The following positions are designed to help make your pregnancy more comfortable by relieving the pressure of the uterus on various parts of your body and by reducing the strain on some of the muscles and ligaments. None of the positions should be maintained for prolonged periods of time since they would not be good for your circulation. Also, when getting up from any of the positions, you should do so slowly, so your won't feel light headed.

Tailor Sitting

Purpose: To allow air to circulate around the perineum.

To shift the weight of the uterus from the back to the front of the pelvis. A comfortable position for pregnancy and labor.

Position: Sit on a carpeted floor or rug with your hips and knees flexed, but don't let one foot rest on top of the other since this position impedes the circulation in your legs. You may rest your arms on your legs.

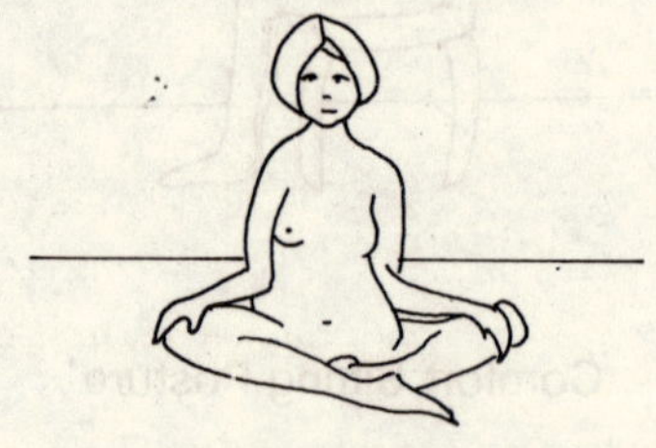

Tailor Sitting

Semireclining

Purpose: A comfortable position to assume for practicing relaxation An excellent position assume if you are having trouble lying on your back because of a light-headed feeling or backache. A comfortable position for labor.

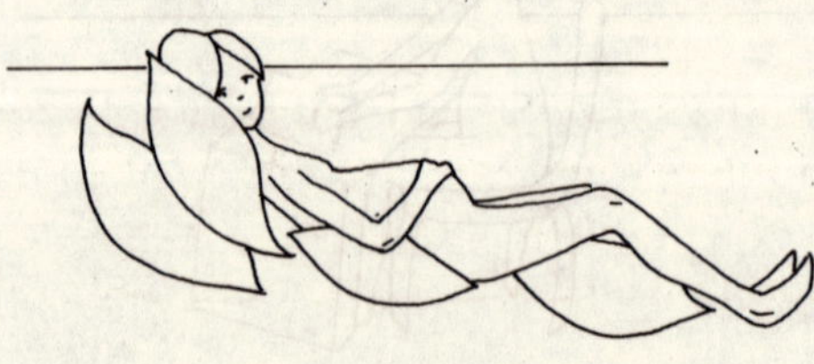

Semi-reclining Position

Position: Lie in a semireclining position. Use pillows behind your head and back to prop you up to a 30 to 40 degree angle.

Side-lying

Purpose:. A comfortable position to assume for sleeping or resting in pregnancy A good position for labor

Position:. Version 1. Lie on your side with lower arm behind your back and the other arm in front of you. Place pillows under your head and shoulders, forward arm, chest, and uterus and one between your legs. Both knees should be drawn up slightly toward your chest with the top leg drawn up higher and ahead of the bottom leg. This is the "runner" position.

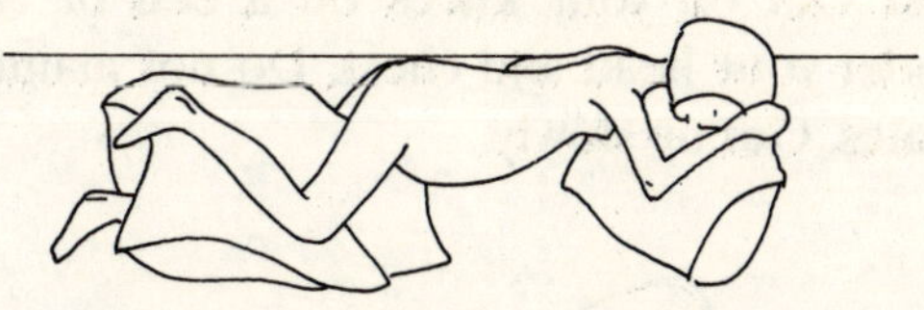

Sidelying in "Runner" Position

Version 2. Lie of your side. Place one pillow under your head and shoulders and several pillows under your lower legs to raise them higher than your hips.

Note: Lying on your side, especially on your left side, is a recommended position for pregnancy because it keeps pressure off the blood vessels behind the uterus while at the same time helping to drain excess fluid from your legs and feet.

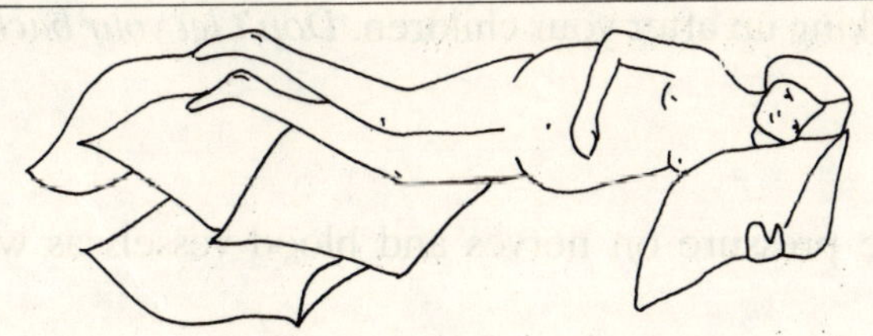

Sidelying Position with Legs Elevated

Back-lying

Purpose:. For some, a comfortable position for sleeping, reading, or relaxing. This position is not recommended for labor because of the increased pressure of the uterus on the inferior vena cava (blood vessel behind the uterus), which can result in a drop in the woman's blood pressure (venous hypotension) and a subsequent faint feeling.

Position:. Lie on your back with a pillow under your head and one under your knees and things.

Note: Do not keep a pillow under your knees for prolonged periods of time as this can impede circulation in your legs.

Using Knee-Chest of All-Fours Position

Purpose:. Takes the pressure of the uterus off the nerves and blood vessels that go to the legs and pelvic organs.

Can help relieve backache, cramps in the groin or legs, vaginal and rectal swelling.

Note: The knee-chest position should not be used in labor.

Positions: Knee-Chest Get on your knees on a bed or carpeted floor. Lean forward, placing a pillow under your head and chest. Do not maintain this position for more than two or three minutes. Get up slowly.

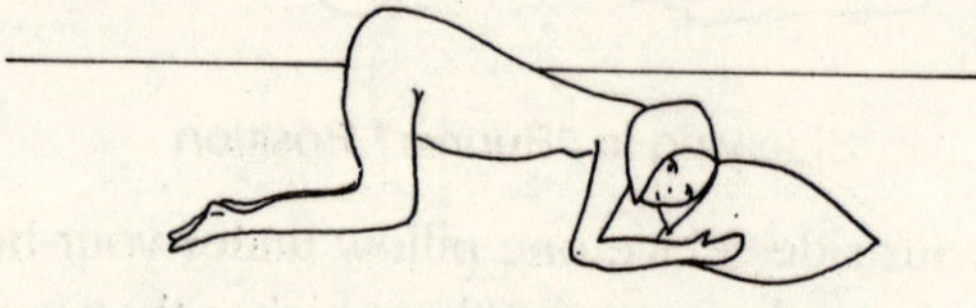

Knee-chest Position

All Fours. Get on your hands and knees with your arms directly under your shoulders and your legs under your hips. This position can be assumed when scrubbing the floor, gardening, or picking up after your children. *Don't let your back sag.*

Elevating Legs

Purpose:. To relieve pressure on nerves and blood vessels as well as on pelvic organs.

To improve circulation and decrease leg swelling.

Position:. Version 1. Assume a leg-elevated, head-down position. Lie on the floor and put your feet up on the couch or low chair. Place pillows under your hips so your entire body is almost straight, not flexed. You should be at about a 30 degree angle. Do not stay in this position for more than 5 minutes at a time and get up slowly.

Position:. Version 2. To promote good circulation while sitting or lying, elevate your legs so they are higher than your heart. Do the sand-digging exercise.

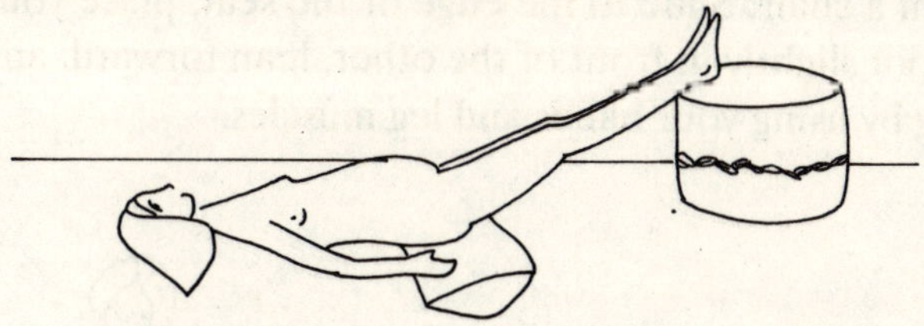

Body Elevation – Backlying with Feet Up

Squatting

Purpose:. The best alternative to bending over when opening drawers, or picking up things from the floor.

Stretches lower back muscles and loosens pelvic joints.

Position:. Unless your legs are strong and you feel stable, squat while holding onto a piece of furniture of other object.

Once down, you can continue to stabilize yourself by keeping your hands on the floor.

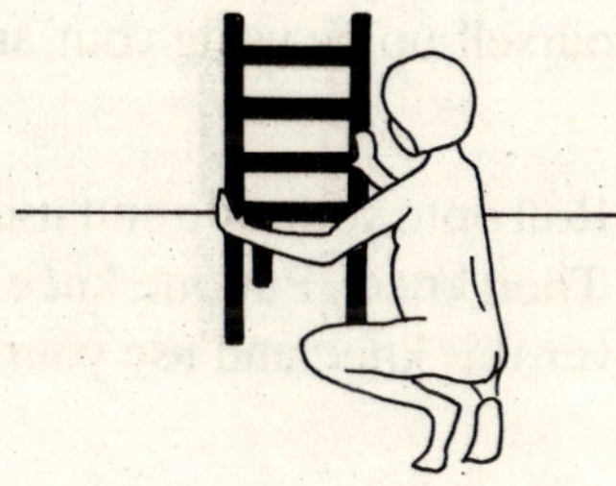

Squatting

To get up, keep your back straight and lift by straightening your knees. Again use something stable to balance yourself as you rise. Do not straighten your knees and then lift up your back from the waist.

If squatting is difficult for you, don't worry about it. You can kneel instead.

Body Mechanics

Practicing proper body mechanics when rising from a bed, a chair, or the floor will prevent strain on muscles and unnecessary stress on your back.

- Rising from a chair: Slide to the edge of the seat, place your feet on the floor with one foot slightly in front of the other, lean forward, and push yourself up to standing by using your hands and leg muscles.

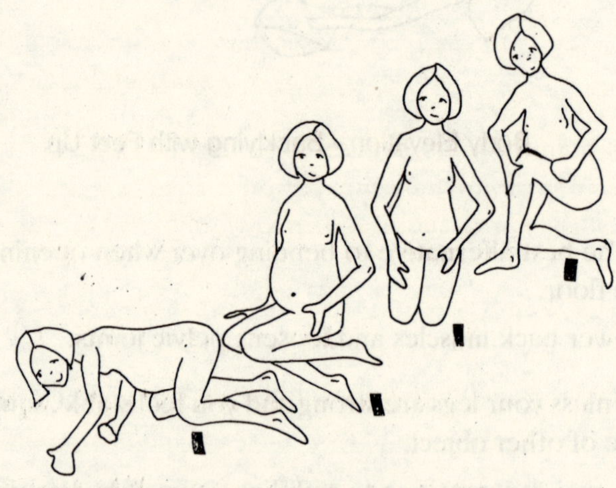

Rising from the Floor

- Rising from bed: Roll over onto your side and swing your legs over the edge of the bed as you raise yourself up by using your arms. Once sitting, continue as above.
- Rising from the floor: Roll onto your side and use your arms to push yourself to a side sitting position. Then kneel. Put one knee in front with your foot on the floor. Bend forward over this knee and use your arms and legs to stand. Keep your back straight.

Prenatal Physical Preparation

Exercises should be an important part of your preparation for childbirth. If you have not begun prenatal exercises, it is not too late to start. Although you may not be able to build a great deal of strength late in your pregnancy, you can maintain tone and stretch muscles in preparation for birth.

Even though you may have been fairly active during your pregnancy, most sports and daily activities don't exercise muscles used during childbirth. An exercise program, as outlined in this chapter, will do the most to insure proper tone and elasticity for these muscles. You may continue to engage in sports you have previously enjoyed unless your doctor advises otherwise. Don't however, take up a new sport that is strenuous or dangerous during your pregnancy. Walking, swimming, and bicycling are good forms of exercise.

You should Exercise During Pregnancy for the Following Reasons

1. To help your body withstand increased stress on muscles, joints, and ligaments.
2. To relieve back strain and improve your posture.
3. To maintain stability in your pelvis; hormonal changes during pregnancy soften fibrous tissue and ligaments in the pelvis to loosen the joints; strong muscles in the abdomen and in the pelvis are necessary to maintain good pelvic stability and good posture.
4. To increase circulation in your legs; pressure of the expanding uterus on blood vessels in the lower extremities decreases circulation.
5. To relieve pelvic and rectal pressure.
6. To stretch and strengthen the muscles needed for childbirth.
7. To renew energy and relieve nervous tension.
8. To strengthen the abdominal muscles so they can support the growing uterus and other abdominal organs; occasionally these muscles are pulled apart in the center of your abdomen during your pregnancy, leaving a gap. If muscles are strong, this problem is less likely to occur or to be severe.
9. To improve your self image and feeling of well being.

There are some muscles that sty relaxed during childbirth and some that contract, or work. During delivery, the upper abdominal muscles will contract to help move the baby down the birth canal, and the lower abdominal muscles and the pelvic floor must remain relaxed. Having exercised the appropriate muscles, your will have the strength and control necessary during childbirth. Your body will also be able to cope with the demands put upon it during labor and delivery if you are in good physical shape.

Having maintained some tone in the muscles, you will regain your strength much faster after delivery. You will also feel better because you are not extremely weak and fatigued. Because you have maintained flexibility in your back and tone in the abdominal muscles, you will be able to resume good posture without any difficulties.

Before beginning the exercise program, you should check with your physician to make sure the exercises are medically acceptable for you. You should try to exercise twice a day if possible, doing each exercise five times and gradually increasing the number of repetitions to ten. Don't exercise just before going to bed because the exercises may be stimulating enough to keep you awake. Also, do not exercise right after eating. Should the exercises result in painful muscles or joints, cut down on the number of repetitions. If any exercise is difficult or painful, eliminate it completely.

Exercise on folded blanket or exercise mat on the floor in a well-ventilated room. Wear loose, comfortable clothing.

The Prenatal Exercises

Assume the position given for each exercise. Inhale during the first part of the exercise and exhale during the last part, except where otherwise stated. Do each exercise slowly, relaxing briefly between repetitions and a little longer before beginning a new exercise.

Pelvic Tilt

Purpose:. To increase strength in your abdominal muscles.

To maintain flexibility in your lower back muscles.

To relieve pressure on the nerves and blood vessels of the uterus, rectum, pelvis, kidneys, and legs.

To prevent or relieve backache caused by increases strain on muscles and ligaments.

To improve posture.

Position:. Version 1 Lie on your back with your knees bent.

Exercise. Tilt your pelvis back by pulling in your abdomen and squeezing your buttocks together. Feel the small of your back flatten against the floor. Don't lift up with your feet. Relax. Repeat. (Arrows show tilt).

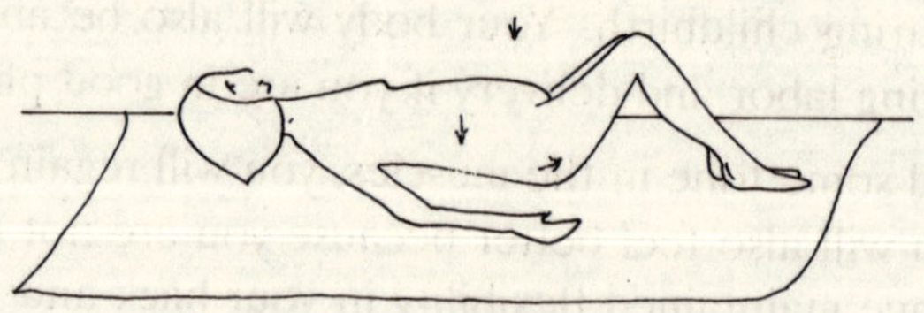

Pelvic Tilt – Backlying Position

Position:. Version 2 Get on the floor on your hands and knees, keeping your hands under your shoulders and your knees under your hips. Keep your back straight; don't let it sag.

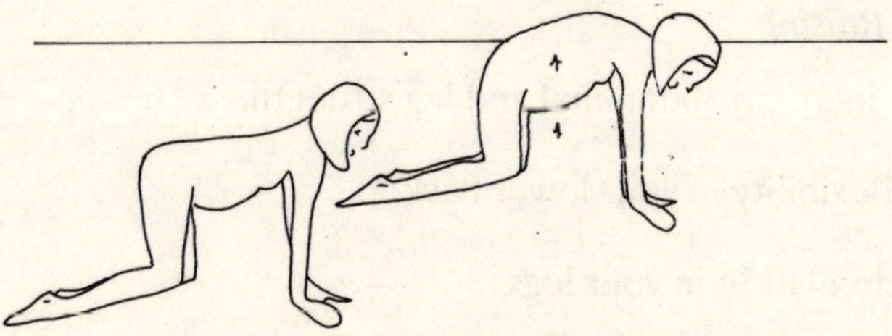

Pelvic Tilt – Hands and Knees Position

Exercise:. Round your lower back by pulling in your abdominal muscles and tightening your buttocks. Your pelvis will tilt backwards as your back arches up. Return your back to a neutral position by relaxing the muscles.

Bridging

Purpose:. To strengthen the back muscles, which together with your abdominal muscles, keep your pelvis tilted back to avoid strain on your back.

Position:. Lie on your back with your knees bent.

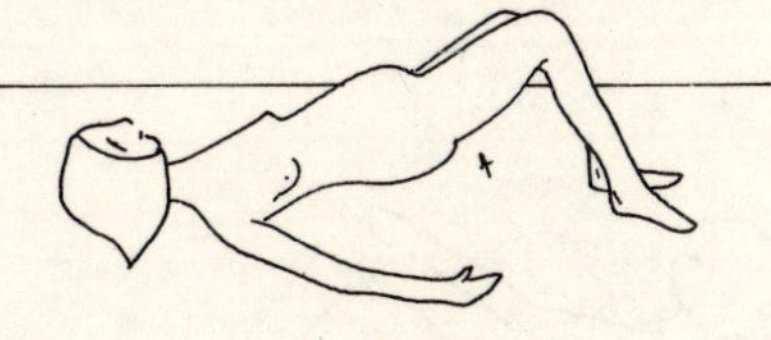

Bridging

Exercise:. Raise your hips off the floor, forming a "bridge." Keep your back straight. Return to the starting position, slowly lowering your back and buttocks. Repeat.

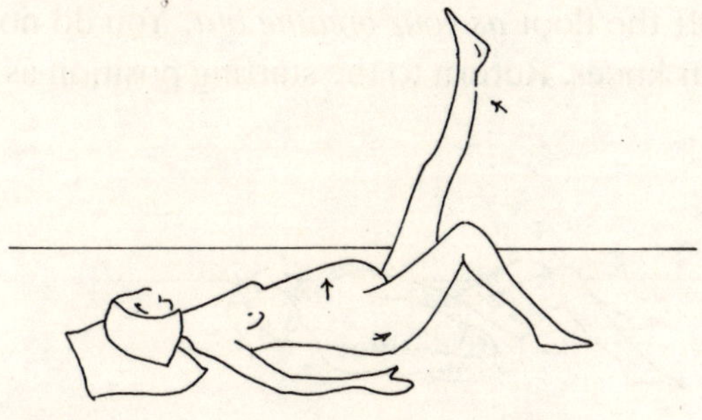

Straight Leg-Raising

Straight Leg Raising

Purpose:. To increase abdominal and leg strength.

To maintain flexibility in your lower back.

To improve circulation in your legs.

Position:. Lie on your back. Bend one knee and keep the other straight. Tit your pelvis back as in the preceding exercise (pelvic tilt, version 1). Maintain the pelvic tilt throughout exercise.

Exercise:. Raise your straight leg up toward the ceiling until the muscles pull behind your knee. Slowly lower the leg, remembering to hold the pelvic tilt. Repeat, raising the opposite leg.

Partial Sit-up

Purpose:. To increase abdominal strength.

Position:. Lie on your back with knees bent and pelvis tilted back. Maintain the pelvic tilt throughout the exercise.

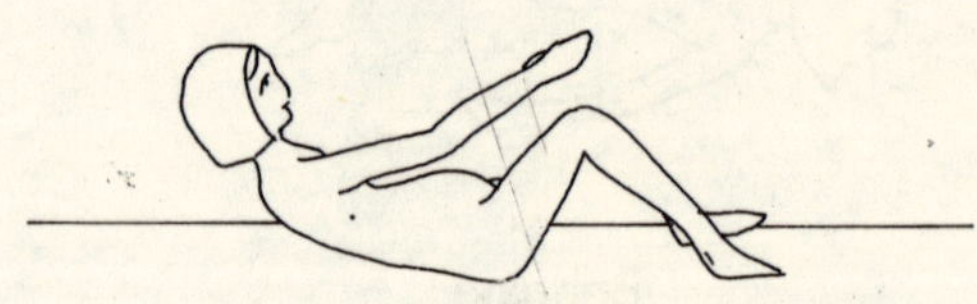

Partial Sit-up – Lifting head and shoulders

Exercise:. Version 1 With your hands outstretched toward both knees, raise your head and shoulders up off the floor *as your breathe out*. You do not need to come up all the way. Do not grab your knees. Return to the starting position as you *breathe in*.

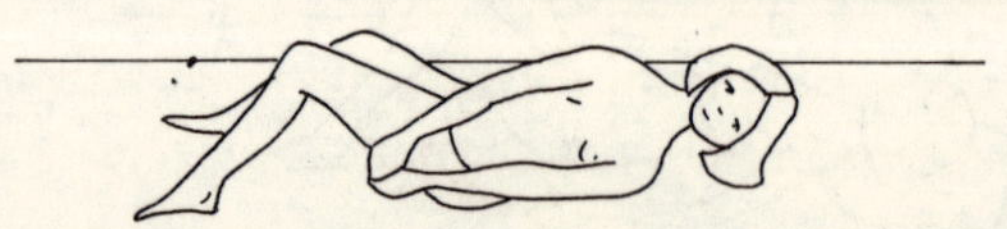

Partial Sit-up – Lifting head and shulders diagonally

Exercise:. Version 2 With both hands outstretched and reaching outside the right knee, raise your head and shoulders up off the floor. (The oblique abdominal muscles are being exercised). Repeat, reaching outside the left leg with both hands. Remember to breathe out as you rise and breathe in as you relax.

Note: If the abdominal muscles separate during the latter months of pregnancy. You will notice a bulge in the center of your abdomen, near the navel, when you raise your head and shoulders straight up (Version 1). Should this problem occur, support the muscles by crossing your hands across your abdomen and pushing the muscles together. Do not raise up very far and do not allow the bulge to appear. Do this a few times during the day to prevent further separation and to maintain tone. Do not do the oblique abdominal exercise (version 2).

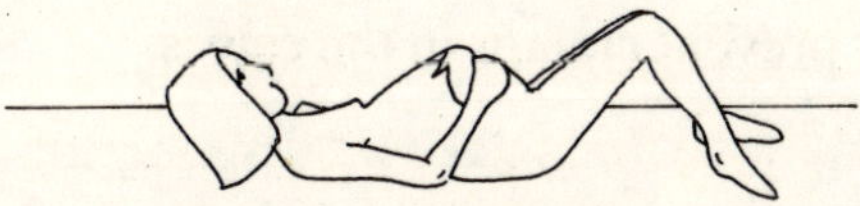

Partial Sit-up – Supporting abdomen with hands

Tailor Stretching

Purpose:. To stretch the inner thigh muscles.

To circulate air around the perineum.

Position:. Sit with your knees bent and the soles of your feet touching. Wrap your arms around the outside of your legs and place your hands just below your knees on the front side of your lower leg.

Exercise:. Push your legs toward the floor, resisting the motion with your arms. Relax, let go of your knees, and use the outer thigh muscles to press your knees further toward the floor.

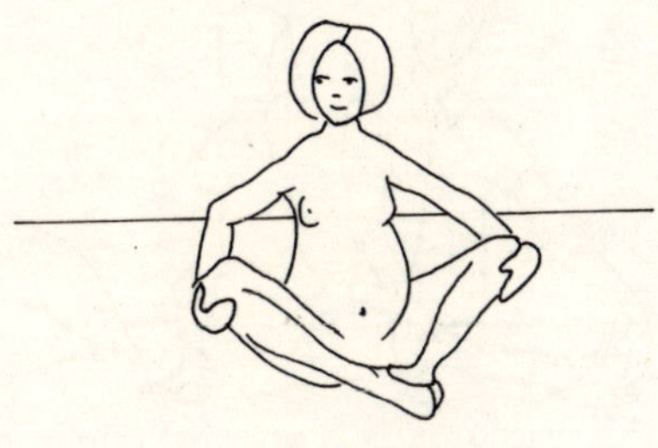

Tailor Stretch

Sand Digging

Purpose:. To improve circulation in your legs.

To help reduce swelling in your feet and legs.

To reduce or prevent cramping and fatigue in your legs.

Position:. Lie on your back with your legs elevated or sit in a chair with your feet up.

Exercise:. slowly make circles with your feet, stretching your ankles in both directions. Imagine that your feet are making circles in the sand at he beach.

Calf Stretching

Purpose:. To relieve or prevent cramps in the calves.

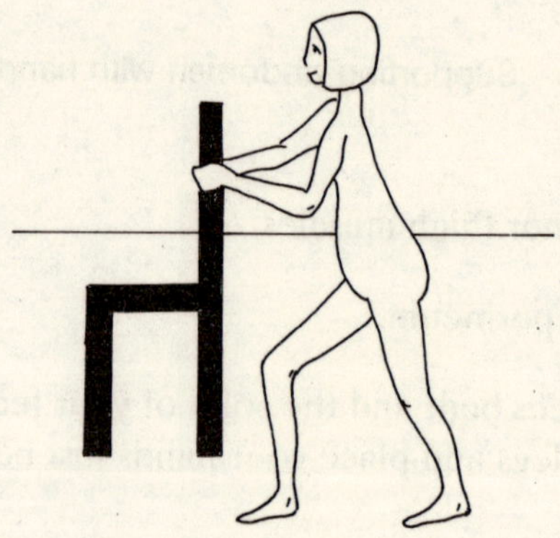

Calf Stretching – Supported by chair with one leg forward, other back

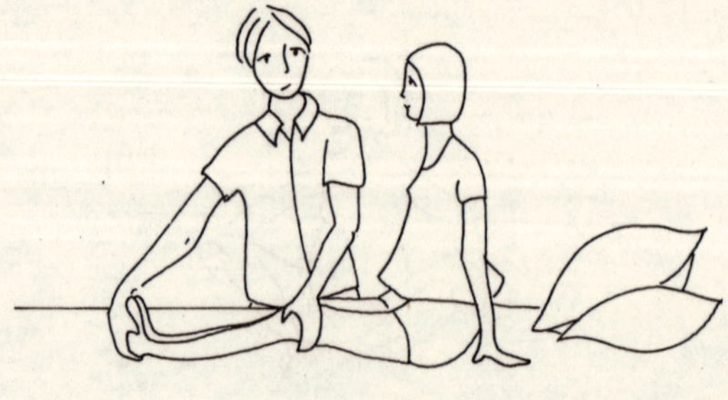

Calf Stretching

Position:. Version 1 Simply stretch the calf muscle by pulling your toes up toward your face. Do this before getting out of bed in the morning and during the day before getting up from a sitting or reclining position.

Position:. Version 2 Stand, placing your hands on the back of a chair or on a counter. Bring the leg with the cramp backward, keeping your heel on the floor. Now bend that knee, getting a good stretch in the calf muscle. The opposite knee will bend too.

Position:. Version 3 Another person can stretch your calf by placing his or her hand under your heel and with the forearm gently pushing your foot up. Your knee should be straight.

Shoulder Circling

Purpose:. To promote better posture by making your conscious of keeping your shoulders back.

To stretch the chest muscles that can cause rounded shoulders if they are tight.

To increase circulation in the postural muscles. To stretch muscles that if tight can impinge on nerves, causing tingling or numbness in your hands and fingers.

Position:. Sit tailor fashion or stand.

Exercise:. Shrug your shoulders up toward your ears; then pull your shoulders back, pinching your shoulder blades together. Return to the starting position and repeat.

Arm Stretching

Purpose:. To expand the rib cage, reducing the discomfort caused by increased pressure in the chest area (helps decrease heartburn, indigestion, and shortness of breath).

To stretch shoulder and back muscles, improving posture.

Position:. Sit tailor fashion or stand.

Exercise:. With both arms above your head, reach up toward the ceiling as far as you can with one arm and then the other. Continue alternating and stretching as far as possible.

Forearm Pressing

Purpose:. To strengthen the muscles under your breasts, thus giving them better support.

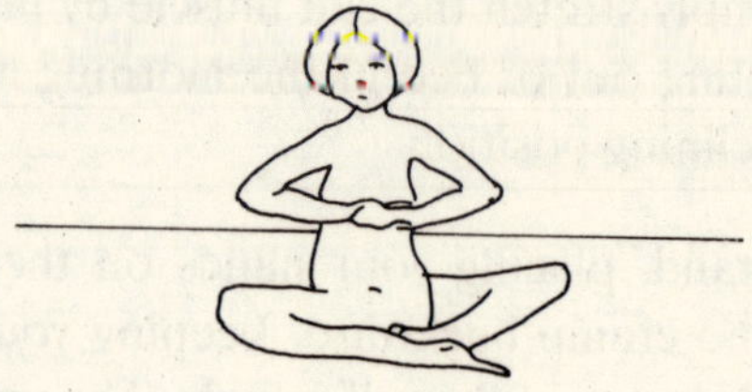

Forearm Press

To increase circulation to the breasts.

Position:. Sit or stand with your arms at shoulder height; bend your elbows and grasp your forearms.

Exercise:. Push your arms in toward each other without letting go of your forearms. Only your skin will move a little. Push and hold to the count of five; repeat.

The Pelvic Floor

The pelvic floor consists of layers of muscles which form a sling across the bottom of the pelvis. The internal muscles act to support the pelvic organs and their contents,

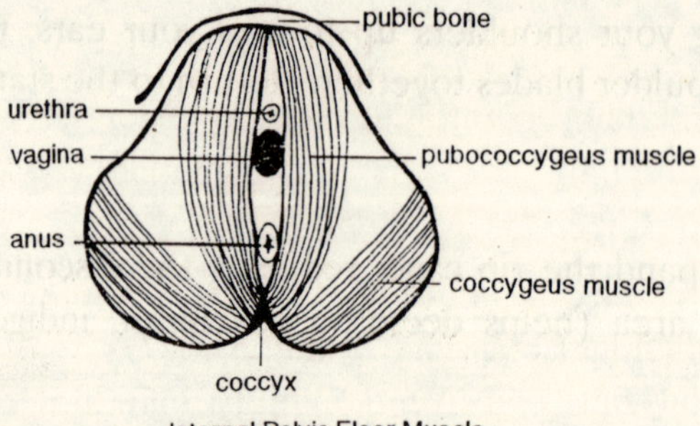

Internal Pelvic Floor Muscle

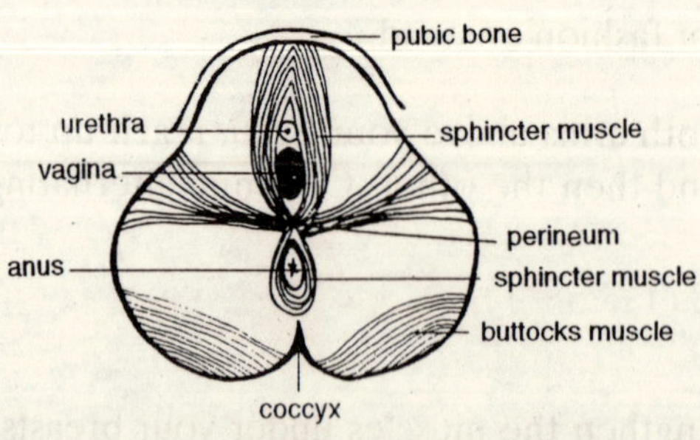

External Pelvic Floor Muscles

and the external, more superficial muscles act as sphincters to open and close the urethra, the vaginal outlet, and the rectum. The pubococcygeus is one of the most important internal muscles. It acts as the primary support for the uterus, vagina, bladder, and rectum. As its name implies, it extends from the public bone in front to the coccyx, or tailbone, in back. While you are pregnant, the pubococcygeus must bear the weight of the growing uterus. During the birth of your baby, it must totally relax to allow passage of the baby's head.

As was mentioned, the pelvic floor muscles support the internal organs, including the growing uterus. As it enlarges during pregnancy, more stress is placed on the pelvic floor, resulting in sagging muscles and loss of tone. Exercising the muscles during pregnancy will help keep them stronger so they can better support the uterus. The birth canal distends more easily and is less likely to be damaged during the birth if the muscles are supple and strong. Also, the pelvic floor exercises help relieve pelvic congestion or swelling during pregnancy and can alleviate or prevent hemorrhoids.

Passage of the baby through the birth canal stretches the pelvic floor muscles even further, resulting in more loss of tone despite your efforts to keep them strong

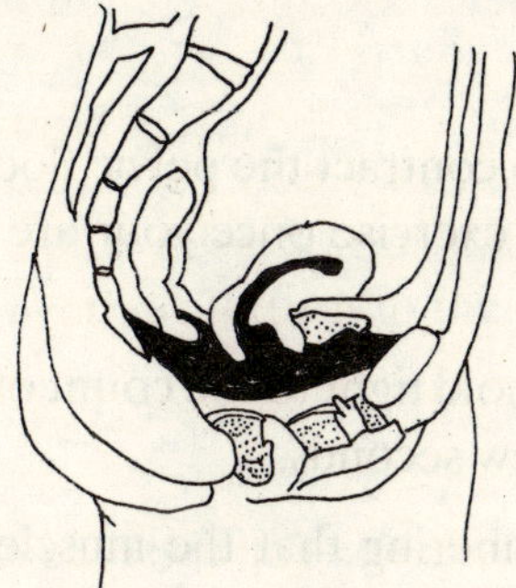

Pelvic Organs – Well-supported by pelvic floor muscles

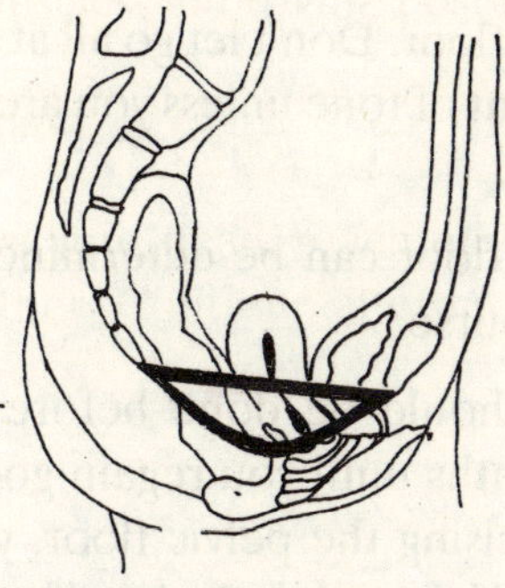

Pelvic Organs – Poorly-supported by pelvic floor muscles

during pregnancy. If you do not continue to exercise the muscles after the baby's birth, loss of tone can result in difficulties. Urinary incontinence is the most frequent problem, which is the inability to voluntarily retain urine when the bladder is full. Laughing, sneezing, coughing, or other stress on the bladder results in involuntary passage of urine. This loss of control can be very annoying or embarrassing if the problem is severe.

Another very important function of the pelvic floor is the tightening of the vaginal canal during intercourse. When the muscles are strong, better contact is made between the vagina and the penis. The resulting stimulation of nerves increases sexual satisfaction.

Doing the pelvic floor exercise immediately after the baby's birth will promote healing of the episiotomy (*see* Chapter Six). Contracting and relaxing the perineum (pelvic floor muscles between the anus and the vagina) helps bring oxygenated blood to the site of the incision and keeps the tissues healthy.

Exercising the pelvic floor after the birth will also prevent prolapse, or sagging, of the rectum, bladder, and uterus. If severe prolapse occurs, the organs may not function well and surgery may be required.

The Pelvic Floor Exercises

- The easiest way to learn to contract the pelvic floor is to stop and start the flow of urine. Discontinue this exercise once your are familiar with the location of the muscles.
- Contract the pelvic floor, hold tight to the count of two, and relax. Repeat. One contraction only takes a few seconds.
- Elevator exercise: Remembering that the muscles are in layers, pretend that you are on an elevator going up Start by tightening the superficial sphincter muscles on the ground floor. As you count to four, contract higher and higher, around the birth canal. Hold tight to the count of two, and then slowly come back down to the ground floor. Don't let go all at once. Your pelvic floor always maintains a certain amount of tone unless you are consciously relaxing it, as you will be during delivery.

The strength of your pelvic floor can be determined by evaluating the pressure exerted on the penis during intercourse.

The pelvic floor exercises should be done before the birth of your baby and continued for several weeks or months until you regain good tone in the muscles. Since nobody is aware that you are exercising the pelvic floor, you can do the exercises anywhere. It will help you remember if you plan to do a few every time you engage in a particular activity—while you are doing dishes, talking on the phone, watching television, or feeding the baby. Immediately after the baby is born, it will be easier to do the exercises lying down because you will be eliminating the pull of gravity on the muscles.

The pelvic floor muscles are not strong like your thigh muscles, for example, and especially after childbirth, will not tolerate excessive exercise. Start by doing five or six repetitions at a time, and if you feel the muscles becoming tired even before then, stop, and next time decrease the number of repetitions. Do these exercises eight to ten times a day. Gradually increase the number of repetitions to ten or twenty. In six or eight weeks you should be able to do about thirty repetitions without difficulty. At this point your muscles are quite strong, and you can stop doing the exercises on such a regular basis. However, always check yourself to make sure you don't lose tone over a period of time.

30

Anatomy and Physiology of Childbirth

You will better understand the changes occurring in pregnancy and childbirth if you are familiar with the anatomy of the mother and baby. It will help you to communicate with your doctor and the hospital staff if you understand the process of childbirth and are familiar with some commonly used medical terms.

Anatomy of Mother and Baby

Uterus

The uterus (1) is a hollow, thick-walled muscle which receives the fertilized egg and houses the fetus as it grows. The uterus is capable of tremendous stretching to accommodate your baby's growth.

The uterus is composed of muscle fibers that are arranged in a lengthwise and circular fashion. Because of this arrangement, the uterus is capable of very powerful contractions, which gradually open the cervix during labor.

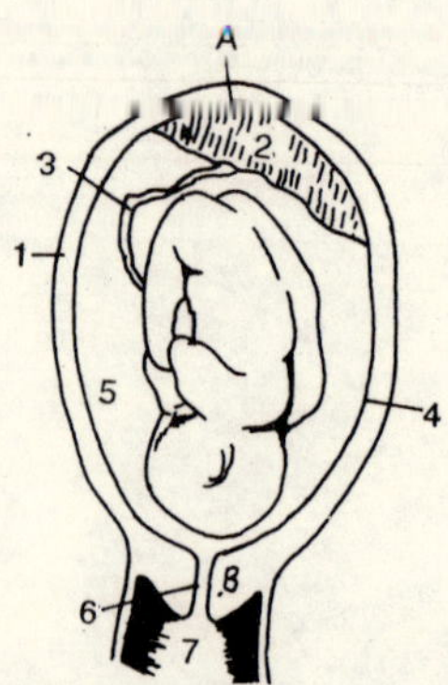

(1) uterus; (A) fundus; (B) cervix; (2) placenta; (3) umbilical cord; (4) amniotic sac; (5) amniotic fluid; (6) mucous plug; (7) vagina (birth canal).

The *cervix* (B) is the thick, closed, bottleneck-like opening to the uterus. During labor it must open enough for the baby to pass into the birth canal. The *fundus* (A) is the upper third of the uterus.

The uterine muscle is an *involuntary* muscle, which means that you cannot control its contractions.

Following delivery the uterus will *involute* or return to near prepregnant size in two to sic weeks.

Placenta

About seven days after conception, the egg (now called an *ovum*) implants in the wall of the uterus and begins to develop into various organs. One of them is called the *placenta* (2). The placenta, or *afterbirth,* functions as an exchanges station between the mother's and baby's bodies. Oxygen and nutrients are supplied by the mother's blood stream and pass through the blood vessels of the placenta to the baby. Carbon dioxide and waste materials from the baby pass back through the placenta to the mother's body to be eliminated. The mother's immunities will also pass to the baby through the placenta. The fetal and maternal bloods do not actually mix. The porous vessels are close to one another, allowing substances to absorb between them.

The placenta does not function as a barrier to keep out undesirable substances, but rather it is more like a sieve. For example, if medication or alcohol are in the mother's system, they also appear in the baby's system. Check with your doctor before taking any kind of medication, including over-the-counter drugs. Research indicates that there are harmful effects on the fetus from smoking, alcohol, and many over-the-counter drugs. *Be very careful what you put in your system when pregnant or trying to get pregnant.* At birth the placenta weighs one pound. Following its delivery, contraction of the uterus helps to control bleeding from its site of implantation. The uterus is very sensitive to touch following delivery.

Umbilical Cord

The umbilical cord (3) is attached at one end to the placenta and at the other end to the baby. It contains two arteries which carry fetal blood to the placenta and one vein carrying fetal blood back to the baby. The site where the cord attaches to the baby becomes the *umbilicus* (navel, or belly button) once the cord has been clamped and cut at birth.

At birth the cord is about two feet long, or the length of the baby. It is filled with a substance called *Wharton's jelly,* which surrounds and protects the cord's blood vessels. Because of the Wharton's jelly and the force with which the blood flows through the cord, it becomes very rigid, helping to keep the cord from knotting and tangling as the baby moves. It is similar to the way a garden hose cannot be knotted when the water is rushing through it.

Because of the length of the cord, it is possible for the baby to become tangled or for the cord to wrap about some part of the baby's body. During pregnancy this occurrence is not a problem. As the baby moves deeper in the pelvis during labor, there may be some strain if the cord is around the baby's neck. Your doctor or nurse would recognize this condition during labor from the pattern of your baby's heartbeat. It is not uncommon for a baby to be born with the cord around his neck, and it is usually not a problem. Once the head is born, the doctor slips her finger under the cord and pulls it over the baby's head.

Amniotic Sac and Fluid

The fetus is enclosed in tough, slightly elastic membranes called the amniotic sac (4). These are sometimes called the *membranes or the bag of waters,* All these terms mean the same thing. The sac acts as a seal to protect the baby from infection. Within this sac is a clear, colorless, watery substance called *amniotic fluid* (5), which serves many functions for the baby. It regulates temperature, is a medium for movement, and cushions the baby from blows. It is completely replaced every three hours. At birth there are usually one to two pints of fluid.

Sometimes during or just before labor the amniotic sac will rupture or tear. You may feel a trickle or gush of fluid and perhaps confuse it with accidental leakage of urine. *It is important that you call your doctor if you suspect that your membranes have broken.* If they are ruptured, it means that the protective seal around the baby is gone, and the baby and you are subject to infection. If the membranes do not rupture on their own, your doctor will probably rupture them either at the end or sometime during your labor. This is a painless procedure.

Mucous Plug

The mucous plug (6) is a protective mass of mucous filling the cervical canal. It helps to protect the baby from infection caused by bacteria in the vagina. As the cervix begins to change before labor, the mucous plug will often be discharged. It looks like a clump of mucous which is blood-tinged or pinkish. It is not a lot of bright red blood. Should you experience this kind of bleeding call your doctor. Sometimes women lose their mucous plug and don't notice it. Its loss is not considered a definite sign that labor is imminent, although it frequently precedes labor.

Vagina

The vagina (7), or birth canal, extends from the cervix to the vulva, or external opening to the vagina. After the cervix is open, the vagina is the canal through which the baby passes. The vagina is very elastic, made more so by the hormones of pregnancy. Because it can easily stretch to accommodate the baby, it does not require contractions to open it up as did the cervix. Toward the end of pregnancy you may notice an increase in vaginal secretions.

Ligaments

Three main ligaments maintain the position of the uterus: the broad, round, and uterosacral. The increase in size and weight of the uterus during pregnancy puts stress on these ligaments and can cause discomfort where they attach in the low back and groin areas.

Uterine Function

If you were to look up "labor" in a medical text, you would read something like this:

The rhythmic contraction and relaxation of the uterine muscle with progressive effacement and dilatation of the cervix leading to delivery of your baby.

But what does it mean? Let's break it down into parts.

Contractions

If you have never had a baby, how do you know what contractions are? Maybe you have felt your abdomen getting tense or hard, then relaxing or softening; or perhaps you have experienced an intermittent backache or menstrual-like cramping above the pubic bone. These are contractions. More specifically, they're called *Braxton-Hicks contractions,* or warm-up contractions. Your uterine muscles have been contracting throughout pregnancy, but you become more aware of it during your last trimester. Usually Braxton-Hicks contractions are not painful, but they may be uncomfortable. Often they occur when you're trying to rest or when you've been standing or walking for a while. Braxton-Hicks are useful because they are preparing the cervix for labor; that is, they are softening or *ripening* the cervix in preparation for the changes that will occur during labor.

Contractions begin at the fundus, or top of the uterus, and radiate over the body of the uterus toward the cervix.

Contractions should be called contractions. *They should not be referred to as labor pains.*

We can draw a picture of a contraction, like the following:

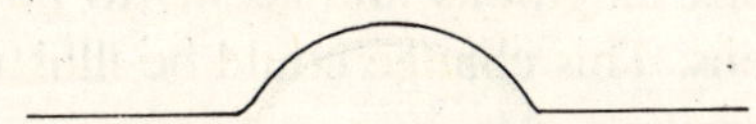

This is a contraction of early labor. It has a gradual buildup in *intensity,* or pressure, a period of greatest intensity called the *apex*, or peak, and then an easing off of pressure.

A series of contractions could be pictured as follows:

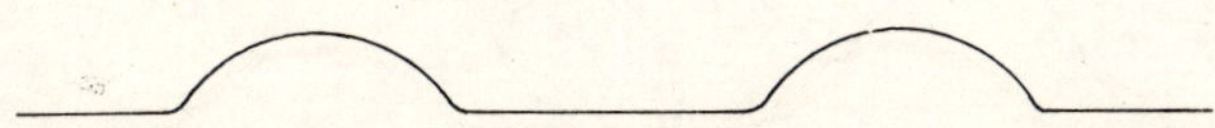

Here you see the rhythmic, wave-like quality of the contractions. You need to know how to talk about contractions. One thing you're interested in is how long the contraction lasts, or its *duration.* You also want to know how often the contractions are occurring, or their *frequency.* The frequency of contractions is measured from the beginning of one to the beginning of the next one. The *interval* is the rest phase between them. For example:

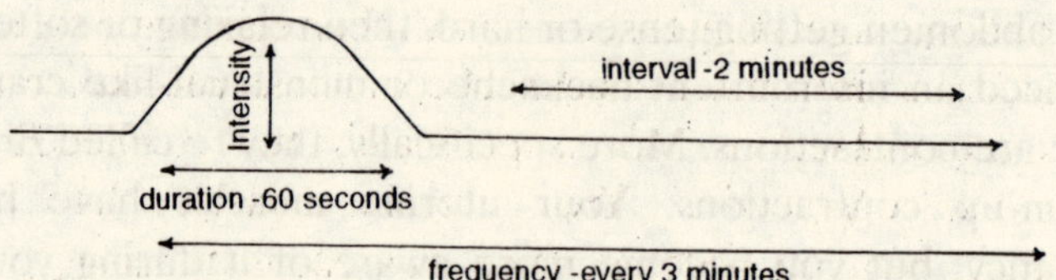

- The *interval* of this contraction is two minutes.
- The *duration* is sixty seconds.
- The *frequency* is every three minutes.
- The *intensity is* a personal evaluation of the strength of the contraction and can be measured with a monitoring device as milliliters of pressure.

As a woman progresses through labor, a pattern usually evolve and her contractions become progressively longer, stronger, and closer together. Because this pattern occurs gradually over a period of several hours, the woman is able to adjust to it.

As labor becomes more active, the quality of the contractions changes; that is, the buildup time shortens, the apex lengthens and seems to be consistently more intense, and the easing-off time shortens. This change could be illustrated as follows:

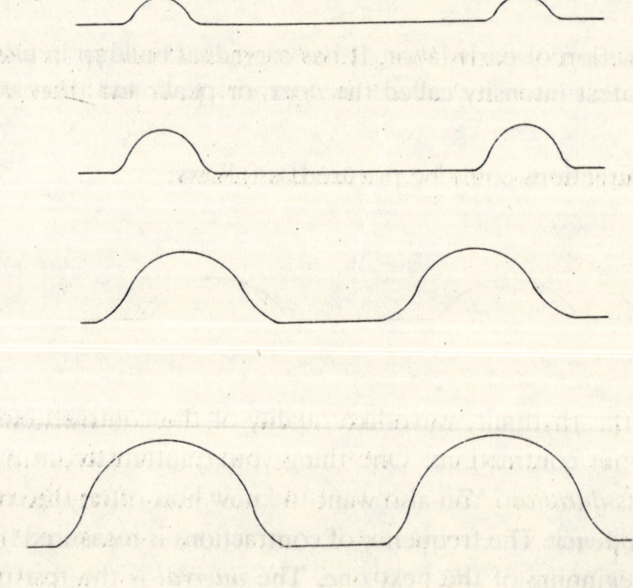

Effacement

The term refers to the thinning of the cervix. When you have a contraction, the lengthwise uterine fibers are *contracting*, or *shortening*, and pulling up the circular fibers around the cervix—which causes the tow-inch-thick cervix to thin out, or efface, until it is paper thin.

Effacement is measured in percentages by your doctor or nurse during a pelvic exam. Complete effacement, or thinning, would be called 100 percent effaced.

If you are having your first baby, most cervical effacement occurs before much dilatation begins. If you are having a second or later baby, the cervix can efface and open at the same time. Sometimes effacement occurs before labor if a woman has a lot of Braxton-Hicks contractions.

Effacement for a primipara, or woman having her first baby, can be shown as follows:

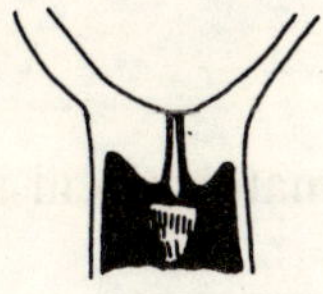

Before Labor Cervix is thick and Closed

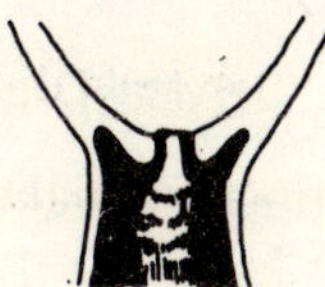

Early Effacement - Cervix is partially effaced

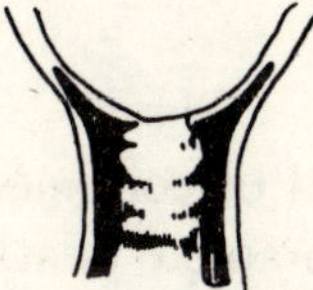

Complete Effacement - Cervix is paper thin Dila - tation has begun

Dilatation

Dilatation is the opening of the cervix to allow the baby to pass out of the uterus and into the birth canal. It is caused by contractions and the pressure of the baby's presenting part—usually the head—on the cervix. As in the case of effacement, dilatation can sometimes begin before a woman actually goes into labor. Dilatation in measured in centimeters, or cm. Complete dilatation is 10 cm, or about 4 inches.

Dilatation can be determined by your doctor or nurse during a pelvic exam. It is a somewhat arbitrary measure, since each person may judge the distance the cervix has opened slightly differently. For this reason, the doctor often says, "You're one to two cm," or "You're five to six cm."

When doing a vaginal exam during labor, your birth attendant uses tow fingers to periodically measure the dilatation of your cervix. You can spread your first two fingers to measure the opening in the chart above. Occasionally dilatation is described by fin-

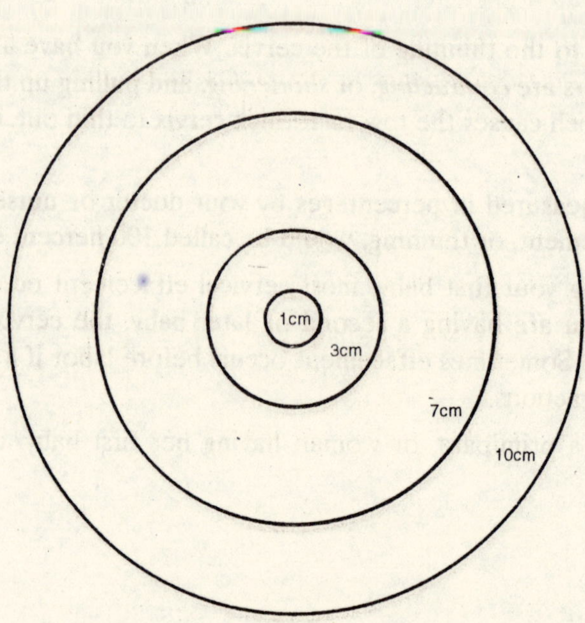

Cervical Dilation

gers instead of centimeters—one finger equaling approximately 2 cm and five fingers meaning complete dilatation.

Dilatation can be illustrated as follows:

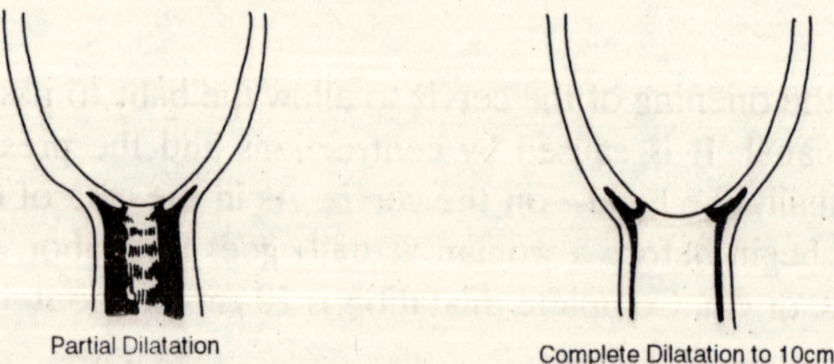

The time during which effacement and dilatation of the cervix take place is called *labor.* when the cervix is 100 percent effaced and 10 cm dilated, it is said to be *complete.* The cervix has opened and been incorporated into the uterus and a funnel-like structure now exists for the baby to make his exit. labor is completed, and the delivery or expulsion stage begins.

Stages of Childbirth

Childbirth is divided into various stages. Labor, one of the stages, is divided into various phases. The chart on the opposite page illustrates the stages of childbirth.

The Maternal Pelvis

The pelvis is made up of four bones—two hip bones, the sacrum, and the coccyx (tailbone)—united at four joints.

These bones are united by fibrocartilage and ligaments. In the front, the two hip bones meet each other to form the *symphysis pubis.* They meet the sacrum at the two *sacroiliac joints,* and the sacrum and coccyx unite to form the *sacrococcygeal joints.*

Early in your pregnancy, your baby is protected within the pelvic cavity, but as he grows, the uterus will grow up and out of the pelvic cavity and then descend again close to your due date or when your go into labor.

Stages of Childbirth

Stage 1 – Labor	(Phases of Labor)
The cervix effaces and dilates.	*Latent or early labor*
	Effacement occurs and the cervix dilates 2 to 3 cm.
	Active labor
	Dilatation progresses from 3 to 7 cm.
	Transition
	Cervix dilates from 7 to 10 cm.
Stage 2 – Expulsion	
The baby moves down the birth canal and is born	
Stage 3 – Delivery of the Placenta	
Delivery of the placenta, or afterbirth, occurs shortly after the baby's birth.	
Stage 4 – Postpartum	
The mother's vital signs stabilize.	
She is carefully monitored during this recovery phase.	

There are several things the doctor wants to know about the relationship of the baby to your pelvis. This relationship will have a direct influence on how you pelvis. This relationship will have a direct influence on how you experience labor and delivery. It is important of you to understand what your doctor is looking for in your last few weeks of pregnancy. If you talk to your doctor, you will have a better understanding of what is happening to your body and what to expect about your labor and delivery. When your doctor or nurse does a pelvic examination, ask about the findings. Stay informed.

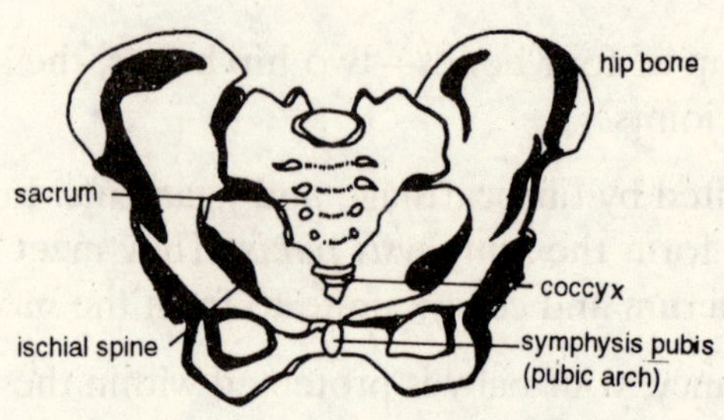

Maternal Pelvis

Size

Early in your pregnancy your doctor measured your pelvis by palpating, or feeling, the bones. He was checking to see that your pelvis can accommodate the average seven-pound baby.

Late in your pregnancy, your pelvic joints relax somewhat. The maternal hormone, *relaxin,* causes the ligaments of the pelvis to soften and become more mobile, allowing it to expand to accommodate the baby. In addition to some give in the mother's pelvis, there is also some in the baby's head. The skull bones of the baby are not yet solidly fused, allowing them to mold during the birth process. The give in the mother's pelvis and the give in the baby's head permit delivery of a normal-sized baby to a woman with a normal pelvis.

If in doubt about the fit, your doctor may request an *ultrasound* or *x-ray pelvimetry* (see Chapter Twelve) to measure your pelvis and the baby's head.

Presentation

Presentation can easily be remembered by asking. "What part presents itself first to the doctor?" About 97 percent of the time the baby's head comes first, giving a *cephalic,* or *vertex,* presentation. In general, the baby's head makes the best dilator of the cervix and the best occupier of the pelvis.

When it is not a vertex presentation, it may be a *breech* presentation. The incidence in about 3 percent. There are different types of breech presentations. In the *complete breech,* the buttocks and legs are born first, and the knees and hips are flexed.

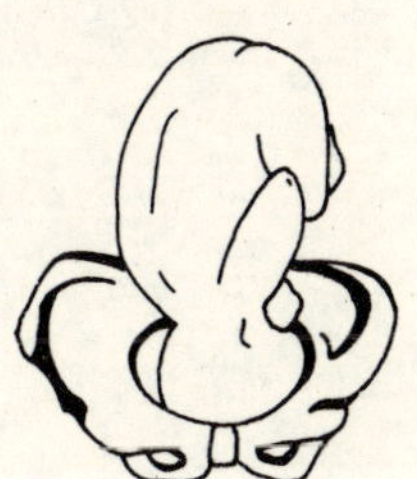

Cephalic or Vertex Presentation

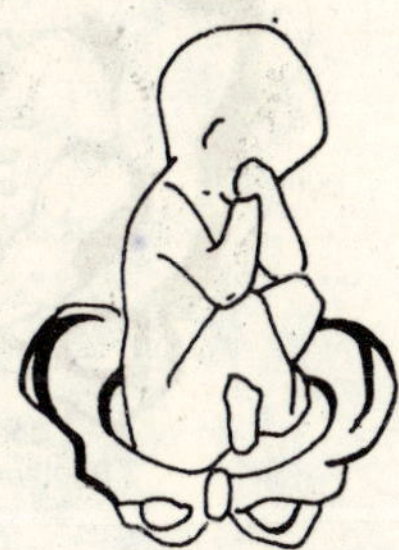

Complete Breech

In the *frank breech,* the buttocks are still first, but the legs are straight and the feet are up by the baby's head.

A *footling breech* can be single or double footling, depending on whether one or both feet are first.

In the *kneeling breech,* the baby is in a kneeling position.

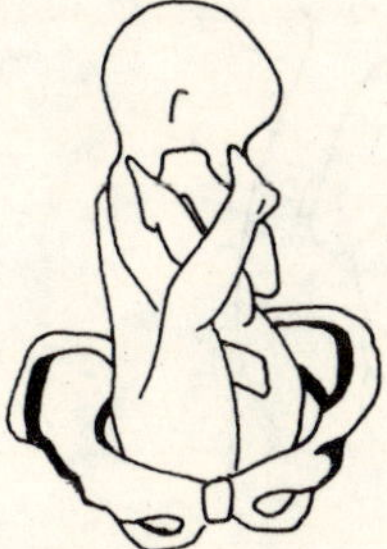

Frank Breech

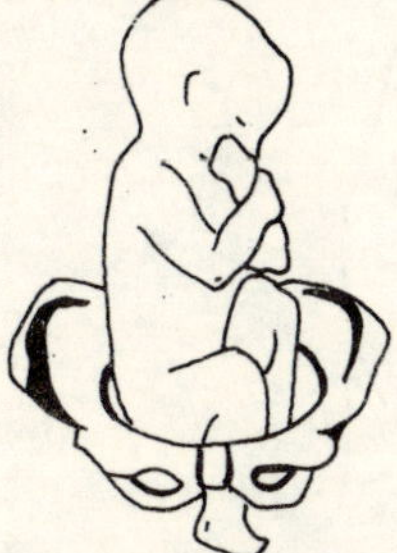

Footling Breech

A third way in which a baby may be presenting is called *transverse lie,* in which the baby is lying across the mother's pelvis. It is not possible for a baby in this position to be born vaginally, and unless the position changes, a Cesarean section will be performed. The incidence of transverse lie is rare.

Position

Position refers to which way the baby is facing in relation to the mother's back. Looking at the mother's pelvis we could label the following directions:

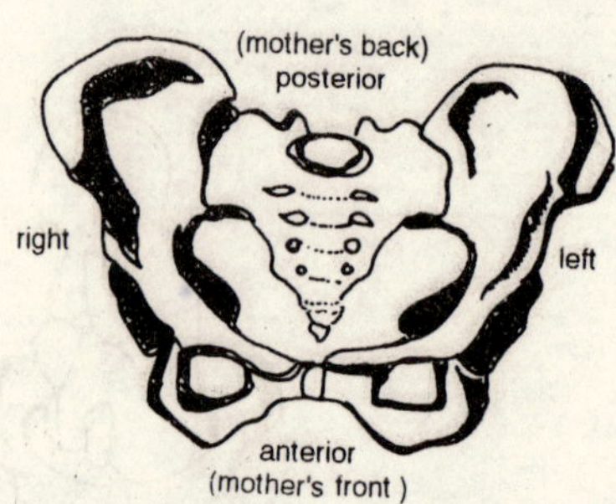

As the reference point on the baby's head, we use the *occiput* or crown. Let's say the baby is arranged in a vertex presentation. He can be anterior or posterior, to the right or to the left. Let's look at each of these positions in more detail to see how they can influence your labor and delivery.

Anterior. If the baby is head down with the occiput toward the mother's front (the baby is looking toward the mother's back), this is the *occiput anterior position*, either right or left. It would be labeled in this manner:

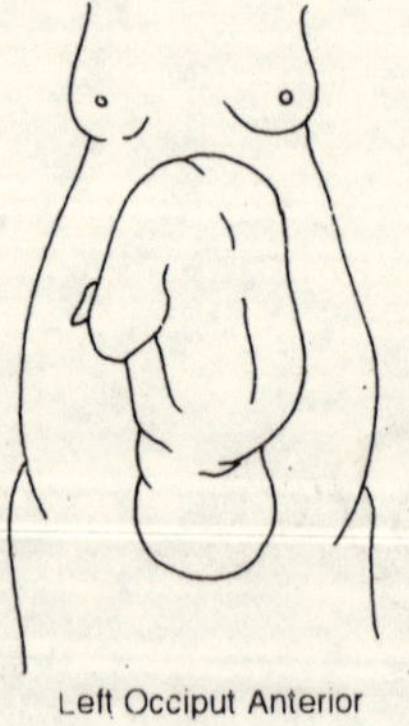
Left Occiput Anterior

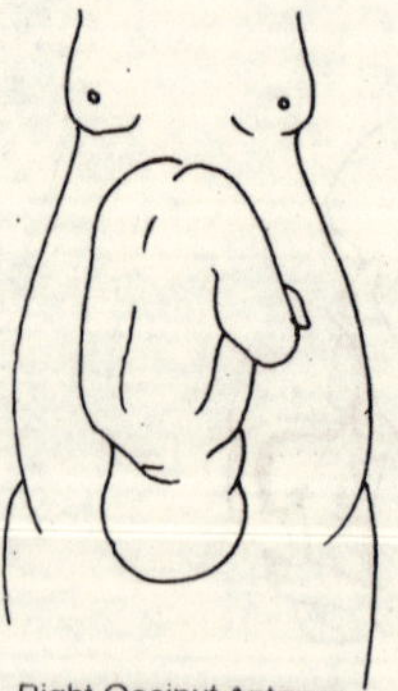
Right Occiput Anterior

The left occiput anterior position is the most common and also the most preferable since it requires the least amount of rotation for the baby to be born. Position is important because of its influence on labor and delivery, and in anterior positions the following labor usually results:

1. The mother is able to lie comfortably on her back with the head of the bed elevated. She may complain of mild backache.
2. The contractions will probably be felt more in the abdominal area and have an equally long and strong pattern.
3. The baby rotates and is born looking toward the mothers back.

Posterior. If the baby is head down with the occiput toward the mother's back (the baby is looking toward the mother's front), this is the occiput posterior position, either to the right or the left.

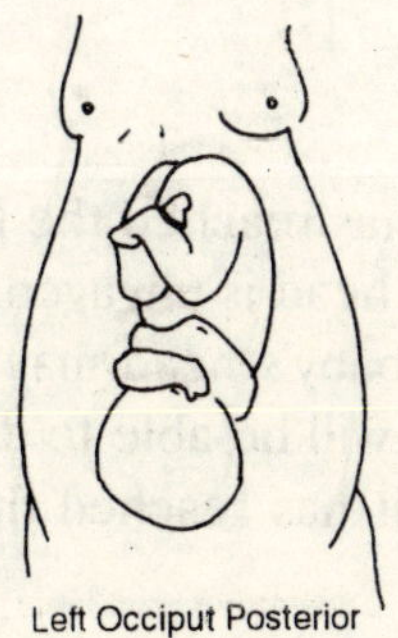
Left Occiput Posterior

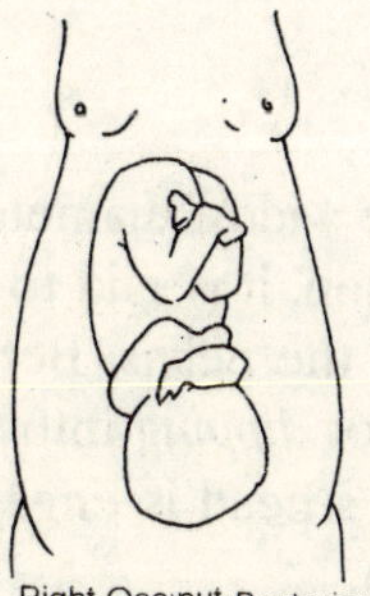
Right Occiput Posterior

The incidence of posterior is about 15 to 30 percent, with ROP more common than LOP.

The following labor usually results from posterior positions:

1. The mother is unable to lie comfortably on her back. She complains about persistent or intermittent backache (see Chapter Ten).
2. The contractions are often irregular—the length, interval, and intensity may vary. The contraction pattern is sometimes one longer, stronger contraction followed by one or two shorter, milder contractions.
3. Contractions are felt mainly in the back rather than the abdomen.
4. There is a longer pushing stage if the baby fails to rotate.

Station

Station describes the vertical descent of the baby into the pelvis, or the amount of downward progress the baby has made. An imaginary line, called *zero station,* is drawn across the ischial spines of the pelvis.

If the baby's head is above the ischial spines it is described as —1 cm, —2 cm, and so on. If the baby's head is below the ischial spines, it is described as +1 cm, +2 cm, and so on. You can remember this designation by thinking that you become positive as the baby moves deeper in the pelvis and you are closer to delivery.

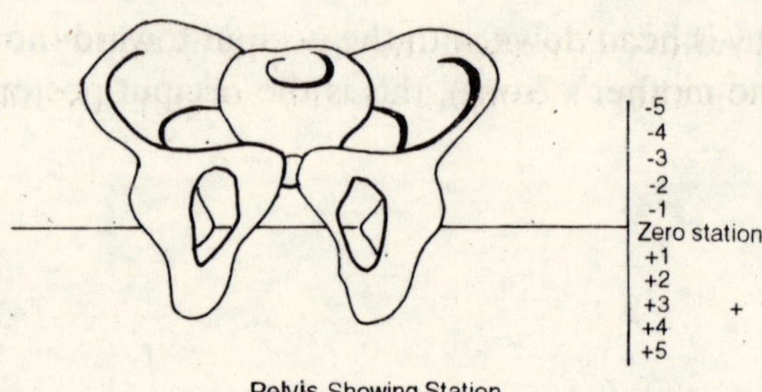

Pelvis Showing Station

When the widest diameter of the baby's head has reached the level of the ischial spines, or 0 station, it is said to be *engaged.* Once the head is engaged, it usually doesn't move up out of the pelvis. Before it is engaged the baby's head may be *floating* above the pelvic inlet or *dipping* into the inlet. Your doctor will be able to determine whether or not the baby's head is engaged and what station it has reached through a pelvic or abdominal exam.

When the baby has descended to the plus stations, the mother may feel the urge to push, the sensation that she needs to bear down to help deliver the baby .

31

Labor

This chapter discusses what happens prior to and during labor. The definition of labor is:

The rhythmic contraction and relaxation of the uterine muscles with progressive effacement and dilatation of the cervix leading to delivery of your baby.

Going into Labor

Labor generally begins when the fetus is able to survive outside the uterus. *Term refers* to the time when the infant has reached the point of maximum intrauterine development, usually 38 to 42 weeks following the last menstrual period (abbreviated LMP). Labor optimally begins 266 or 267 days following conception, or 272 to 280 days following the LMP, or approximately 40 weeks. "Nine months" is misleading. One way to predict the due date is Naegle's Rule: To the first day or your LMP, add seven days and then subtract three months.

Most doctors would agree that it is not easy to predict accurately when labor will begin. Many babies are not born on their due date, or estimated date of confinement (EDC). At best your doctor can estimate whether the cervix appears favorable for labor to begin.

When labor begins before 37 weeks of gestation, the baby is said to be *premature*. There may be some concern about how well prepared the infant is to withstand the rigors of labor and delivery, and then to function independently of the mother.

When labor has not begun by 42 weeks of gestation, the baby is said to be *postmature*. Here, the main concern is whether the placenta is still functioning adequately and whether the baby's source of oxygen and nutrients is being compromised. Your doctor can perform estriol tests to determine placental functioning (see Chapter Ten).

Special precautions are sometimes taken when a laboring woman is giving birth to a premature or postmature infant, which may include decreased medication or anesthesia for the woman and special arrangements in the delivery room (equipment, pediatric personnel, and so on).

Many different theories exist regarding what causes labor to begin, such as ovarian hormones, placental hormones, volume of the uterus, size of the infant, strength of the cervix, or a signal from the fetus. To date, however, there is not a definitive answer to this intriguing, sometimes exasperating, question.

The Length of Labor

Both the mother and the labor coach are concerned about how long it will take to have the baby. Emanuel A. Friedman, a physician, has compiled statistics and arrived

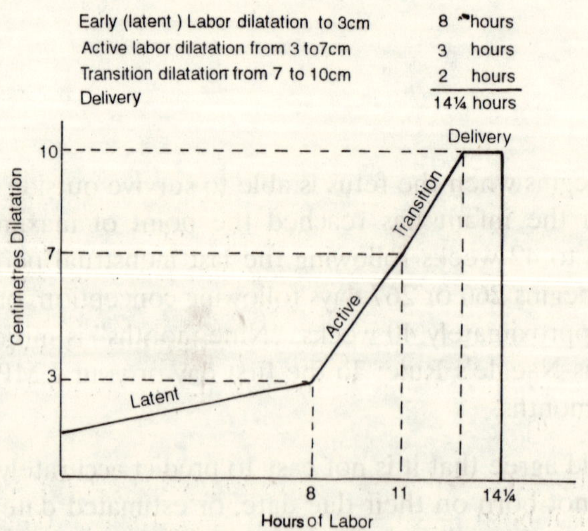

Friedman's Labor Curve for a Primapara

at average times for labor. He has plotted these on a graph, which we have adapted below. The curve shows the progress of an average first labor. Keep in mind that the baby can be born much more quickly than this average, and also, that it can take longer.

Centimeters of dilatation are plotted vertically on the graph, and the number of hours of labor is plotted horizontally. The curved line represents the progress of the *average* labor for a first baby.

In general, your doctor likes to see a primipara dilate at least one centimeter per hour during the active and transition phases of labor.

Prelude Phase

Sometimes women experience a prelude phase, which is an indefinite period—a couple of weeks or days—prior to labor. Many changes may occur during this time. You may feel excited, apprehensive, and irritable. You may be feeling uncomfortable because of the large size of your uterus, and you are feeling very *ready* to have your baby.

During these weeks *it is important of the mother to get plenty of rest.* She should make a concerted effort to be ready for labor. If she is well rested she will find that labor is easier to handle and recovery is more rapid. For a while, your new baby will be getting up for night feedings, so it will not be as easy to get the sleep you need once he is horn.

The final weeks of pregnancy are sometimes hard on both the mother and father. It is helpful for the mother to have as much diversion as possible, without fatiguing herself. She may want to continue to work or spend time with her friends. Now is a good time to splurge on an evening out and doing some nice things: get a new haircut, go out for lunch with a friend, enjoy your baby showers, make something special for yourself or the baby.

Fathers can help by seeing that the mother gets extra rest, by helping her practicc breathing and relaxation techniques, and by reassuring her. Try not to allow yourselves to get discouraged if the due date comes and goes. Massage and back rubs will be appreciated. Labor and those early postpartum days will also be easier for the father if he approaches them well rested.

It may seem as if you're going to be pregnant forever, but these last few days and weeks will pass.

Changes Prior to Labor

To help you recognize your progress during the last weeks of pregnancy, here is a summary of changes you may notice. Not all women will experience all of these.

1. *Lightening and engagement:* This is the process in which the baby moves deeper into the mother's pelvis. it occurs as the lower uterine segment begins to soften, allowing the baby to move lower in the uterus, and as relaxation of the pelvic ligaments allows more room for the baby. This change can occur two to three weeks prior to labor for a primipara, and a few hours or days prior to or during labor for a multipara. you may know this change has occurred because it becomes easier to breathe but more difficult to walk gracefully. At the same time you may notice you need to urinate more frequently and urine may occasionally leak because of weak pelvic floor muscles. You may also notice pressure or discomfort where the uterine ligaments attach in the groin, as well as increased pressure in the lower abdomen.
2. *Ripening of the cervix:* The cervix softens and begins to swing forward to an anterior position. During a vaginal exam, the cervix is much easier to reach than previously.
3. *Loss of the mucous plug:* This is a blood-tinged mucous discharge sometimes called "bloody show." It sometimes occurs but may go unnoticed by the woman.
4. *increased vaginal secretions.*
5. *Backache:* There may be occasional backache because of the increased weight of the uterus pulling on uterine ligaments attached to the lower back and relaxation of the pelvic joints.
6. *Braxton-Hicks contractions:* Warm-up contractions or episodes of false labor may occur and may help begin effacement and dilatation of the cervix.
7. *Weight:* There may be stabilization of weight or loss of one to three pounds.
8. *Diarrhea:* Softer stools or diarrhea are sometimes noted a few days prior to labor.
9. *Rupture of membranes:* A leaking or gush of amniotic fluid may occur if the membranes rupture. This clear, odorless fluid is sometimes difficult to distinguish from urine. Call your doctor if you suspect your membranes are leaking, and be sure to report the color of the fluid. Testing with Natrazine (litmus) paper can determine whether the fluid is urine of amniotic fluid. The vagina is usually acidic and becomes neutral or alkaline when amniotic fluid is present.
10. *Spurt of energy:* This change is meant for labor, not for spring housecleaning.
11. *Nesting instinct:* The woman may become involved in getting everything ready for the baby.

True and False Labor

One question that usually causes anxiety for the pregnant couple is how to know when true labor begins. A common fear is to arrive at the hospital only to find that the labor has stopped; everyone worries about being sent home to wait for true labor to start. Another fear is that delay of the hospital trip might result in delivery in the car or at home. *Many* couples worry about whether they can tell true labor from false labor.

Your doctor and the hospital staff have seen a lot of false labor. Even women who have already had children can go to the hospital in false labor, because it is sometimes very difficult to tell the difference until after the fact, when cervical dilatation has occurred. One woman can be in true labor and only moderately aware of the contractions, whereas another can be in false labor and find contractions quite strong. If you go to you doctor's office or the hospital in false labor, don't be embarrassed or upset, and try not to be too discouraged.

The following are a few guidelines for distinguishing true from false labor:

True Labor	*False Labor*
The contractions:	The contractions:
1. Regular pattern	1. Often irregular pattern
2. Become closer, stronger, longer	2. Can vary
3. Walking increases intensity	3. Changing position may stop them
4. Early contractions rarely exceed 60 sec. duration	4. May last 35-45 sec., or longer than a minute
5. Often accompanied by backache	5. May have backache
6. Hot bath, heating pad, or alcoholic drink will not stop them	6. Heat or alcohol may stop them
The cervix:	The cervix:
Ripens, effaces, dilates	May ripen and show minimal effacement and dilatation
The baby:	The baby:
Starts to descend in the pelvis	May or may not descend in the pelvis

Stage 1: The Labor Process

We have already given an overview of the childbirth process. We now need to look at each of the phases of labor in more detail.

Early Or Latent Labor

This is usually a lengthy phase with slow progress. Uterine contractions are generally manageable.

Progress of cervix

Effacement of the cervix.

Dilatation of the cervix to 3 cm.

Contractions

Length:. A range or 20 to 60 seconds, but usually 30 to 45 seconds long.

Interval:. Every 20 minutes, working their way down to every 5 minutes, is usual. However, it is possible that your contractions may not start out at 20-minute intervals but may be either further apart of closer together.

Time: 6 to 8 hours is common for the first labor; however, it may be shorter or longer.

Intensity: Short, mild contractions, with a generally mild apex—gradual increase in pressure and gradual easing off of pressure. Long rest phase between contractions. Contractions get progressively longer, stronger, and closer together.

Physical Signs That May Occur

- Loss of the mucous plug.
- Rupture of the membranes of continued leaking of the membranes.
- Contractions may be felt in the lower back or in the abdomen.
- Increased frequency of urination because of the engagement of the baby's head.
- Constipation because of the slowing of digestion.
- Increased vaginal discharge.
- Increased pelvic pressure because of the descent of the baby.
- Menstrual-like cramping.
- Cramps in hips or legs.

Emotional Signs That May Occur

The mother's behavior reflects the energy and excitement she feels about being in labor.

- Ambivalent and anxious until the question of true versus false labor is settled.
- Excited, energetic—relief that labor has begun.
- Very optimistic and confident—assured of her ability to handle labor. Seems to be very independent and self-motivated.
- Talkative, vivacious, spontaneous.
- Feels that things are progressing faster than they really are.

The Mother's Role

1. Maintain your activity. If labor starts at night, try to get more rest. If labor starts in the day, engage in a light, relaxing activity. In other words, don't go to bed, but don't decide to go grocery shopping, clean the refrigerator, or work overtime.
2. Take a shower if someone is home with you. Don't take a bath (your membranes may be ruptured) unless your doctor says you may.
3. Use distraction to get through these early hours of labor: watch television, go to a movie (if your doctor agrees), or play cards.
4. Urinate frequently. A full bladder is uncomfortable and can impede the descent of the baby's head.
5. Don't eat anything hard to digest because labor causes digestion to stop. If your doctor approves, have a light diet, similar to what you would have after stomach flu: Jello, bouillon, tea with honey, ginger ale, toast, and so on. Do not eat any milk products.
6. Call your doctor according to his instructions.
7. Use this initial phase as a time to assess your own particular kind of labor: Where do you feel the contractions? Are they regular? How are they affecting you? Experiment with the techniques and positions you've learned.
8. Begin active relaxation if you feel the need.
9. Begin the first level breathing only when you feel the need.

The Coach's Role

1. If labor starts in the night, try to get some more sleep. Conserve your energy. You'll need it for the harder, later stages of labor.

2. Early labor is the time for you to take care of such things as eating a good meal, making arrangements to miss work, getting some rest. Later, it will be too hard on the mother if you have to leave her for these reasons.
3. Assess the situation and stay clam. Evaluate how the contractions are affecting the mother. Note what positions she seems to prefer and what techniques seem to help. Note any physical symptoms you want her to report to the doctor. Keep track of the frequency, duration, and intensity of the contractions.
4. Help the mother conserve energy, become comfortable, and stay relaxed. Massage may be helpful. Help her with breathing patterns, and stay with her while she showers or gets ready for the hospital.
5. Enjoy this early phase of labor. Share her excitement that labor has begun and your baby will soon be born.
6. If rupture of the membranes occurs, reassure her; she may feel embarrassed.
7. Prepare for the trip to the hospital. Extra pillows for comfort and a large waterproof pad or bath towels are helpful in case the membranes rupture.
8. Work together to make decisions about the mother's care.

Active Labor

The speed of cervical dilatation increases. Contractions, which are more intense, more frequent, and last longer, require more control by the mother.

Progress of cervix

- Dilatation of the cervix from 3 to 7 cm. 100 percent effacement.

Contractions

- Length:. Usually 45 to 60 seconds.
- Interval: May start as far apart as 7 minutes. Toward the end of this phase, may be every 2 minutes. Every 3 to 5 minutes is usual.
- Time:. 2 to 3 hours is common for a first labor; however, this time can vary.
- Intensity: Longer, more intense contractions with longer, stronger apex. Shorter rest phase. Contractions get progressively longer, stronger, and closer.

Physical Signs That May Occur

- If your membranes are still intact, they may rupture spontaneously or be ruptured by your physician. Remember that contractions can be irregular following rupture and then will usually fall into a pattern of longer, stronger, closer contractions than before. Ask the doctor if your membranes need to be ruptured for medical reasons or if they can be left intact; laboring with intact membranes is usually more manageable.
- Contractions may be irregular and more intense following a pelvic exam.
- There may be discomfort or pressure in your hips and legs due to the pressure of the baby descending deeper into the pelvis.
- There may be nausea and/or vomiting.
- There may be backache.
- Involuntary reactions to stress may appear, such as an increase in respirations, heart rate, and perspiration.
- There may be muscle tension.

Emotional Signs That May Occur

The mother's behavior reflects the increased intensity of the contractions and her fatigue from dealing with them.

- Less talkative and sociable.
- Less aware of environment; more serious; more involved in the labor and dealing with the contractions. Needs to concentrate.
- Still interested in medical details concerning her progress—results of pelvic exams, observing contraction pattern on monitor tracing, if a monitor is used, and fetal heart tones.
- More dependent on her coach, doctor, and medical staff. Loses feeling of independence.
- Needs frequent encouragement.
- Begins to need strong coaching.
- Toward the end of this phase she may become worried about her ability to handle contractions.

The Mother's Role

1. Be sure to catch each contraction at the beginning. Avoid dozing or napping between contractions; you may be caught unaware.
2. Use intervals between contractions for maximum relief and rest.
3. Change position frequently; avoid lying on your back. Try lying on your left side or sitting propped in a bed or chair.
4. Use first-level breathing as long as possible, changing to second-level breathing only when you must. Use second-level breathing when apex of contraction becomes more difficult.

The Coach's Role

1. Coaching becomes increasingly important to the mother. Assess how labor is affecting her and try to help where she is having a problem. Actively coaching her through a contraction by breathing with her may be important at times. She will benefit more from being reminded about techniques rather than having to recall them. Remind her to have a focal point, stay relaxed, and use the appropriate breathing pattern.
2. Breathing pattern should be rhythmic, consistent in speed, and as slow as possible. Watch for signs of hyperventilation and help her correct her breathing pattern if necessary.
3. Watch or gently touch all body parts to check for signs of tension. Use touch and massage to relax specific body parts.
4. Use all available techniques for comfort: ice chips or popsicles cold cloth for neck or brow position change effleurage and petrissage back massage fresh gown, pad, or sheets blanket warm socks straightened bed sheets extra pillows.
5. Sit down sometimes during her labor so that you don't become too fatigued.
6. Keep her informed of her progress.
7. Help minimize the distractions around her—glaring lights, noise from the hall, loud voices, and so on.
8. Encourage, encourage, encourage; praise, praise, praise.
9. Get ready for the transition phase of labor. If your must leave your mate, be sure to ask the nurse to coach her.
   a. Change into delivery (scrub) clothes.

b. Get a bite to eat if hungry.

c. Go to the bathroom.

Transition

Transition in a difficult period before complete dilatation of the cervix. Progress is usually rapid, but there may be a slowing down around nine cm. You may be checked and told that there is still a "rim" of the cervix remaining. Because of the strength and frequency of contractions and some accompanying physiologic and emotional symptoms, transition is usually described as the hardest part of labor; but it is usually the shortest.

Progress of cervix

Dilatation of the cervix from 7 to 8 cm to 10 cm.

Contractions

- Length: 60 to 90 seconds.
- Interval: Variable, usually 30 to 90 second rest period between contractions.
- Time: For average first labor, 30 minutes to 2 hours. The time can vary.
- Intensity: Contractions seem to consist mainly of apex with little buildup or easing off. There may be more than one apex.

Physical Signs That May Occur

- Increased rectal pressure due to descent of the baby; may feel pressure or discomfort in hips, legs and buttocks.
- Nausea and possible vomiting, especially near 10 cm.
- Shaking, trembling legs.
- Urge to push as the baby moves deeper tin the pelvis; may occur before cervix is completely dilated.
- Fatigue and drowsiness.
- Cold feet caused by poor circulation as the baby moves deeper in the pelvis.
- Backache or feeling of pressure in the back.
- Leg cramps.

- Chills, shivers, or a feeling of being overheated; alternately hot and cold; perspiring.
- Continued leaking of membranes and bloody show.
- Loud, long burping.
- Restless; unable to find a comfortable position.

Emotional Signs That May Occur

The mother's behavior reflects the very stressful contractions and her fatigue.

- Uncooperative and demanding; may verbally express these feelings. You may be ungrateful, despite your coach's attempts to help you.
- Panicky, especially if you lose control during a contraction and feel you won't be able to get through it.
- Discouraged—may cry; may say you can't continue.
- Very inward—totally involved with yourself and what's happening to your body; loss of interest in progress of labor and baby. May not be interested in participating in decisions about your care.
- Confused, disoriented; not as aware of environment and things happening around you. May have to be told something several times before you really hear it. Unable to concentrate.
- Very dependent on the coach and staff. You may panic if your coach leaves the side of the bed to stretch his legs between contractions or lets go of your hand. May get upset if your doctor or nurse leaves the room, even momentarily.
- May feel trapped by the relentless quality of the contractions and the feeling that you aren't in control of your body. May say you've had enough and want to go home.
- May project some of the feelings you have to those around you, coach or staff. May verbally snap at them.
- Extremely sensitive to touch; external fetal monitoring belts, effleurage, back massage, wrinkles in the bed sheets, and so on may really irritate you.
- may question the reason for certain medical procedures and feel that nobody understands what you're experiencing.
- Loss of inhibition; personal modesty decreases; less cautious about what you say.

After reading this list of possible symptoms, you may wish that you did not have to go through transition.

Keep in mind that these are possibilities for all women in labor, and that no one woman will experience everything mentioned.

Transition is hard, but it is the shortest phase of labor for most women; and soon you will begin pushing and the baby will be born.

The Mother's Role

1. Concentrate on getting through one contraction at a time. With strong coaching and encouragement from those around you, you can work through each contraction and handle this phase of labor. Transition is hard work, but it can be managed.
2. Transition contractions are very strong and may no longer fit into the pattern established earlier in labor. Don't be upset or alarmed by their strength, frequency, or irregularity. These contractions are normal for transition. Don't be afraid that something has gone wrong with you or the baby. Strong contractions in transition are good; they are dilating your cervix.
3. Try to express any needs you have with which the coach or staff can help you, for instance, if you're cold or hot or want to change your positions.
4. Relaxation in most difficult during transition but should be one of your main tasks. Don't think that you're doing the techniques incorrectly because you're having trouble getting through the contractions. Labor, especially transitions, is hard work; these techniques help control contractions but do not eliminate them.
5. Try not to give in to any panicky feelings about the contractions but to accept them as the mechanism that is causing your cervix to open enough to allow the baby to pass through. Visualize the cervix opening up more and more with each contraction.

The Coach's Role

1. Don't leave her. Be sensitive to how dependent she is and to how much she needs you.
2. Strong coaching is helpful; use simple directions and declarative statements. Be firm, quiet, and assured. Don't ask questions that require more than a yes or no. Take one contraction at a time. Help her stay alert between contractions. Make

sure she's ready for each contraction and starts the breathing pattern right away. Remind her to relax and keep her focal point

3. Adopt a thick-skinned attitude. Do not react to any "abuse" you may receive. Don't take it personally, even if she says it's all your fault. Some of the things she gets angry about may not seem to be rational, but don't argue with her.
4. Do not react to any panic or discouragement she shows. Be reassuring and supportive. Don't you panic. She's looking to you for support and encouragement, not sympathy.
5. Do not react negatively to anything she may do, such as crying or vomiting, or if she doesn't act as you thought she would. Don't have expectations about how your mate will react to labor before it happens. Transition is really hard, and she's never been through it before. No one knows ahead of time how it will be and how one will react.
6. When she's voicing discouragement or saying that she can't continue she's really asking for encouragement and support. Saying she can't do it doesn't necessarily mean that she wants you to agree with her. Tell her she's doing a good job; help her with the breathing; tell her the baby's almost here and soon she can start pushing. Do anything that seems to relieve her anxiety.
7. Be affectionate; praise her; give her lots of encouragement.
8. Stay close to her. She may want to use your face as her focal point. Be ready to breathe with her through a difficult contraction. Though she may be very sensitive to touch, she may still want you to hold her hand or be near her so that she feels you're physically helping her through the contractions and won't level her alone. Continue to encourage relaxation, especially in her shoulders.
9. Be a screen from any disturbing things going on in the labor room. Remember she may be supersensitive to strong stimuli—lights, noise, conversations, someone bumping into her bed. Try to correct any of these situations if they seem to be bothering her.
10. Don't be embarrassed or intimidated in front of hospital staff about being a good coach. If you need assistance or suggestions, the staff is there to help you.

What You should Take to the Hospital

You will want to have things ready to take to the hospital a few weeks before your due date. You don't need to take the clothes you and the baby will wear home from the hospital, but put them where your mate can find them easily to bring to you.

Suitcase

When you are admitted to the hospital, you will be taken to a labor room. Find out beforehand whether or not your suitcase goes with you or if it is put in your postpartum room. You may want to pack a bag of things you will need in the labor room and leave your suitcase locked in the trunk of your car until you are in your postpartum room.

Articles needed for Labor

Chapstick or Other Lubricant for Your Lips

Once admitted to the hospital you probably will not be given anything to eat or drink, and your lips can become quite dry. Some doctors allow their patients to have ice chips or popsicles.

Unscented Powder, Cornstarch, or Lotion for back Rubs and Effleurage

Massage will be much more effective with some lubrication.

Warm Socks

A must, even in July. Toward the end of labor the circulation in your legs may be impaired as the baby moves deeper in the pelvis. Cold feet can be quite uncomfortable.

Hard Candy

If you want to take along hard candy, get the sour, not the sweet, version. Candy on a stick can be easily taken out of your mouth before a contraction begins. Ask if your doctor approves of hard candy for energy and to wet your mouth during labor.

Paper Bag

This is to breathe in if you should hyperventilate, though a surgical mask is as effective and much less cumbersome. Tell your nurse if you need one. Take the beg in case you can't get a mask right away.

Small Hot Water Bottle

For backache. Find out if your hospital provides one if you need it.

Watch with a Second Hand

In case there is no clock in the labor room. Check on this during your tour. Is it where you can see it?

Camera and Film

A flash may not be acceptable in the delivery room if combustible gases are stored there. Check when you go on your hospital tour. If you cannot use a flash, you will need to use high speed film such as Kodak's Kodacolor 400 CG 135.

32

Planning Your Pregnancy

Pregnancy is a major event. When it is planned in advance, a woman can make decisions that will benefit both her health and that of her baby. Good general health before pregnancy can help you cope with the stress of pregnancy, labor, and delivery. It can also help ensure that neither you nor your baby is exposed to things that could be harmful.

Many women do not know they are pregnant until 5, 6, or even 8 weeks. About 2 weeks after a woman's menstrual cycle, an egg can be fertilized by a man's sperm; it them moves to a woman's uterus and becomes attached there to grow. These early weeks are some of the most significant ones for the baby, because it is during this time that the baby's body and internal organs are formed. Certain substances—for example, alcohol, cigarettes, and drugs—may interfere with that growth, whereas a healthy life style may help promote it. Preconception, or prepregnancy, care can guide you in planning for a healthy pregnancy.

A Preconception Visit

You may wish to arrange a special visit with your doctor to discuss your plans for pregnancy. As part of your preconception visit, you will be asked questions about your medical history, any past pregnancies, and your life style. The answers to these questions should be honest and open. They will let your doctor know whether you may need special care during pregnancy, and they will be treated as confidential information.

Some women have medical conditions that require special attention or care during pregnancy. The condition may be an illness that was present before pregnancy or it may arise during pregnancy.

Because pregnancy puts special demands on a woman's body, a health problem that is normally under control can change while you are pregnant. Certain medical conditions, such as hypertension and diabetes, should be brought under control before you become pregnant and may require more frequent visits to your doctor or other special attention. Changes in your life style may also be in order, and your doctor may be able to offer suggestions for improving it.

If you've had a problem in a previous pregnancy, that doesn't necessarily mean that the problem will recur or that you shouldn't try again. Some problems develop a pattern of repeating, but most do not. If a problem is apt to be repeated, you should be aware in advance that you may need special attention before and during your pregnancy.

If you have a family history of birth defects, your doctor may suggest that you see a genetic counselor. Genetic counseling can also help identify a pattern of inherited disorders, if one exists. Common genetic disorders and the way they are inherited.

Your preconception visit is a time for you to ask questions, too. Don't hesitate to ask for advice or discuss any concerns you might have. Your doctor is there to provide information and guidance.

Diet and Weight

A balanced diet is a basic part of good health at all times in your life. The foods you eat are the main source of the nutrients for your fetus, the term used to refer to the baby while it is growing inside you during pregnancy. As the fetus grows and places new demands on your body, you will need more of most nutrients than you did in the past. A good prepregnancy diet is the best way to ensure that you and your fetus start out with the nutrients you both need.

your body functions best when it is well fueled with a balanced diet. To choose that diet, you should be aware of what nutrients your body requires, how much of each nutrient you need, and which foods are good sources. Healthy eating practices are not just for pregnancy, but for the rest of your life. An appropriate healthy diet can easily be modified during pregnancy to provide the extra calories you need. Nutrition in general and the extra needs of pregnancy are discussed later.

Special Diets

Your doctor may detect needs in your diet that should be met before you become pregnant. The factors listed below can affect how your body uses nutrients. If any of these factors apply to you, consult your doctor, because you may need to change your diet.

- Do you take medication (prescription or over-the- counter) regularly?
- Do you follow a strict vegetarian diet?
- Do you run long distances or perform strenuous exercise on a regular basis?
- Do you fast?
- Do you follow a reducing diet?
- Do you have a history of anemia?

Phenylketonuria is an inherited condition that keeps the body from processing an essential amino acid found in foods that contain protein. As a result, the levels of this amino acid build up in the mother's body and can cause birth defects and mental retardation in the fetus. If you were treated for phenylketonuria, probably as s child, you still have the disorder, even if there are no signs of it. However, by following a special diet before pregnancy, you can help keep this condition from affecting your baby during pregnancy, even though there is still a small chance that the baby will inherit the disorder. Before trying to become pregnant, you should consult a doctor and be following a special diet if you have phenylketonuria.

Weight

Every woman would like to maintain an ideal weight for her height. If you're planning to have a baby, however, it's important that you not be excessively underweight or overweight before pregnancy. Underweight women tend to have smaller babies. This is not an advantage, however, because smaller babies have more problems during labor and in the nursery. In general, being overweight is a health hazard. During pregnancy, being overweight is linked to having high blood pressure or diabetes. Extreme obesity puts a strain on the heart that becomes an added burden during pregnancy. Women who are overweight are also more prone to discomforts during pregnancy. It is not a good idea to be on a weight-loss diet while you are pregnant or trying to become pregnant, however. This type of diet could deny you and your baby the nutrients you both need. The best way to plan for your pregnancy is to try to reach an ideal weight before you become pregnant. You will be more comfortable during pregnancy, and the extra weight you gain will be easier to lose later.

Overweight or Overfat?

Fat is the form in which energy is stored. If a diet provides excess calories, they are stored as fat. Obesity is having too much fat. It is difficult to define exactly when a person goes from being slightly fat to being obese. A standard method is to compare a person's body weight with the "ideal" weight for someone who has the same height and frame. If you weigh over 20% more than this weight, you are obese.

Body weight is not always a good measure of the amount of fat you have, though. A person who exercises loses fat and builds up muscle, which is heavier than fat. So a physically fit person can have a body weight that is above normal, but an amount of fat that is below normal. By contrast, a person who is not very active may weigh just as much as a physically fit person, but the inactive person will have more fat and less muscle. Generally, it is normal for a woman to have up to 20–25% of her total body weight in fat.

*Height and Weight for Women**

Height		*Weight (lb)*		
Feet	*Inches*	*Small Frame*	*Medium Frame*	*Large Frame*
4	9	99–108	106–118	115–128
4	10	100–110	108–120	117–131
4	11	101–112	110–123	119–134
5	0	103–115	112–126	122–137
5	1	105–118	115–129	125–141
5	2	108–121	118–132	128–144
5	3	111–124	121–135	131–148
5	4	114–127	124–138	134–152
5	5	117–130	127–141	137–156
5	6	120–133	130–144	140–160
5	7	123–136	133–147	143–164
5	8	126–139	136–150	146–167
5	9	129–142	139–153	149–170
5	10	132–145	142–156	152–173
5	11	135–148	145–159	155–176

*Height shown is without shoes, and weight is without clothes.

Exercise

Good health at any time in your life depends not only on proper diet but also on getting enough exercise. What you can do in sports and exercise during pregnancy depends on your health and, in part, on how active you are before you become pregnant.

When beginning a program, decide whether you want to improve your heart and lung function, the tone of your body muscles, or both. Then, select exercises that will enable you to meet your goals. If you are not used to being active, you should begin an exercise program gradually.

Exercise to improve your heart and lung function can be measured by keeping track of your heart rate. When you know how your heart rate responds to exercise, you can find out how hard to exercise. You should exercise so that your heart beats at your target heart rate, because this is the level that gives you the best workout.

Your Target Heart Rate

To find your target heart rate, look for the age category closest to your age and read across. For example, if you are 29, the closest age on the chart is 30; the target heart rate is 114–142 beats per minute. Your maximum heart rate is 220 minus your age. Your target heart rate is 60–75% of the maximum. These figure are averages to be used as general guidelines.

*Target Heart Rate of Nonpregnant Women**

Age (years)	*Target Heart Rate (beats per minute)*	*Average Maximum Heart Rate (beats per minute)*
20	120–150	200
25	117–146	195
30	114–142	190
35	111–138	185
40	108–135	180
45	105–131	175

*National Heart, Lung, and Blood Institute. Exercise and your heart. NIH Publication No. 81–1677. Washington. DC: U.S. Government Printing Office, 1981.

Every time you exercise, you should begin with a 5- to 10-minute period of light activity, such as brisk walking, as a warm-up before each session. Once your body is warmed up, exercise for 20–30 minutes at your target heart rate. After this 20–30 minute period, you should have a cool-down period of 5–10 minutes. During this period, you gradually reduce your activity, allowing your heart rate to return to a near-normal level.

A program for toning muscles usually requires exercise at least three times a week. It does not have to be done daily—some people's muscles cannot withstand hard exercise every day. Every other day is fine. But it is important that you maintain your routine throughout the year. If you stop for 6—8 weeks, you will need to start again at a lower level of exertion, as if you are just beginning a muscle-toning program.

Cigarettes, Alcohol, and Drugs

Tobacco, alcohol, and drugs are addictive and can harm both you and your fetus. They can have bad effects on the fetus at a time when organs are forming, causing damage that can last a lifetime or even result in death.

Used in combination, as these substances often are, they are even more dangerous. For the sake of your own health and that of you baby, now is a good time to quit or at least cut down your use of tobacco, alcohol, and illegal drugs. By quitting, a pregnant woman helps not only herself, but also her fetus.

It takes time and patience to quit a habit. This is especially true if you've had that habit for a long time. Don't be embarrassed. Ask for help. Your doctor can offer support and medical advice. He or she can also suggest ways to get through the withdrawal stage of quitting. Your decision to quit may be one of the most difficult things you've ever done, but it will be one of the most worthwhile.

Stopping Birth Control

Birth control pills regulate your menstrual cycle. Once you've stopped taking them, your periods may be irregular for a while. This can make it difficult to detect your fertile times, as well as your due date when you become pregnant. Using birth control pills before you become pregnant does not cause any birth defects, regardless of how close to conception you stop using them.

If you have been using an intrauterine device (IUD) to prevent pregnancy, it should be removed before you try to conceive. It is thought that the IUD works by preventing the egg from being fertilized, but pregnancy can occur with an IUD in place. If pregnancy occurs with the IUD in place, it can be harmful; therefore, it should be removed right away by a doctor.

Environment

Some substances found in the environment of at the work place can make it more difficult for a woman to become pregnant or can harm the fetus of a pregnant woman. If you are planning to become pregnant, you may wish to look closely at your work place and environment. If you see that you could be exposed to a harmful substance, then you can take steps to avoid it (see "Harmful Agents,").

Before you accept a job, find out from your employer whether you might be exposed to toxic substances, chemicals, or radiation. Talk to the personnel office about maternity leave, medical benefits, and disability coverage. Once employed, discuss your level of exposure to specific substances with your employee health division, personnel office, or union representative.

Radiation, an invisible form of energy transmitted in waves, in used in some jobs. It is also used to diagnose and treat disease in the form of X-rays. Exposure to high levels of some kinds of radiation can affect the fertility of men and women, as well as affect the fetus of a pregnant woman.

Women planning a pregnancy who are exposed to ionizing radiation in industrial and medical settings should ask for monthly readings of the amount of radiation to which they have been exposed. The amount of radiation received in a chest X-ray, for instance, will not hurt fertility or a fetus. When radiation is used to treat disease such as cancer, however, it is used in much larger amounts and can be harmful.

Exposure to chemicals such as lead, certain solvents, or certain insecticides can reduce your partner's fertility by killing or damaging his sperm. Unlike women, who are born with their complete supply of eggs, men produce sperm most of their lives. Unless the damage to a man's reproductive system is very serious, he will probably be able to produce healthy sperm again a short time after his exposure to the dangerous material stops.

Some pesticides can also damage a woman's eggs, but not as much is known about the effects of chemicals on eggs.

Vaccination

Infection with measles, mumps, or rubella during pregnancy can cause serious birth defects or illness in the fetus. Some vaccines to prevent these diseases may also be harmful to the fetus.

Your doctor may want to ensure your immunity before pregnancy—either by vaccination, documentation of previous exposure, or testing. If you have never had these diseases or do not think you have been vaccinated against them, your doctor may suggest that you be vaccinated before you become pregnant. The vaccine should be given at least 3 months before you try to conceive. During that time you should be using a method of birth control.

If you plan to travel to areas where you may be exposed to infectious diseases not found in this country, you may need to be vaccinated against these diseases. If you are not using birth control, consult your doctor regarding possible effects during pregnancy.

Sexually Transmitted Diseases

Diseases that are transmitted through sexual contact—sexually transmitted diseases—come in all types and forms. Sexually transmitted diseases not only can affect your ability to conceive but can also infect and harm your baby.

The use of some contraceptive methods, such as condoms and spermicides, can lower the risk of getting a sexually transmitted disease. Couples trying to conceive will not be using these forms of contraception. Therefore, they may be at higher risk of getting a sexually transmitted disease if they have more than one sexual partner.

If our think you may have a sexually transmitted disease, see your doctor right away for the appropriate test and treatment. Your partner should also be treated, and you both should abstain from any sexual intercourse until you have completed treatment.

Chlamydia, Gonorrhea, and Pelvic Inflammatory Disease

Chlamydial and gonorrheal infections are the most common sexually transmitted diseases in the United States today. It is thought that about 20–40% of all sexually active women have probably been exposed to chlamydia at some time. People who have or have had gonorrhea are more likely to have a chlamydial infection as well, because the two diseases often travel together.

Chlamydial and gonorrheal infections can cause pelvic inflammatory disease, or PID. This is a severe infection that spreads from the vagina and cervix through the pelvic area and may involve the uterus, fallopian tubes, and ovaries.

The fallopian tubes, through which an egg travels from the ovary to the uterus, also may become scarred and blocked. If this happens, a woman may not be able to have children. In cases of prolonged or repeated pelvic infection, surgery may be needed to remove damaged reproductive organs.

How Sexually Transmitted Diseases Can Affect You and Your Baby

Disease	*Symptoms in Women*	*Effects On:*	
		Mother	*Fetus/Baby*
AIDS	Appetite or weight loss, fatigue, swollen lymph nodes, night sweats, fever or chills, persistent diarrhea or cough	Immune system damage, leading to infections (such as pneumonia) or cancers; death	Immune system damage leading to death in 1–7 years in most infants
Chlamydia	Genital burning or itching, vaginal discharge, painful or frequent urination, pelvic pain; may be no symptoms	Pelvic inflammatory disease ectopic pregnancy	Eye infection, pneumonia
Gonorrhea	Vaginal discharge minor genital irritation; most women have no symptoms	Pelvic inflammatory disease, infertility, arthritis	Eye infection in left untreated
Genital herper	Flu-like symptoms (fever, chills, muscle aches, etc.); small, painful, fluid-filled blisters on genitals or buttocks	Recurrent outbreaks	Severe skin infection, nervous system damage, blindness, mental retardation, death
Genital warts	Possible genital itching, irritation, or bleeding; warts may appear as small, cauliflower-shaped clusters	Warts grow in size and number, cancerous changes	Warts may block vaginal opening
Syphilis	A painless open sore called a chancre; later rash, sluggishness, or slight fever	Damage to heart, blood vessels, and nervous system; blindness, insanity, death	Miscarriage, stillbirth, syphilis in liveborn infant

Gonorrhea and chlamydia can infect the fetus as it passes through the vagina during delivery, causing eye infection and other complications. A newborn's eyes are very sensitive to gonorrhea, and blindness may result. To help prevent this, the eyes of newborns are treated at birth. This is done for every baby whether or not the mother has a history of gonorrhea.

Men with chlamydial and gonorrheal infections commonly have the symptom of a drip from the penis. Many women have no symptoms and find out they have chlamydia or gonorrhea only when their sexual partners are found to have the disease.

Sometimes a pelvic exam is not enough to confirm a diagnosis, and other tests may need to be performed. If you have these diseases, you can be treated with drugs that are safe to take during pregnancy.

Herpes Simplex Virus

Genital herpes is an infection caused by herpes simplex virus. It produces sores and blisters on or around the sex organs. It is transmitted during sexual activity through direct contact with a person who has active sores. Some people have only one outbreak; others have repeated bouts. Although it is rare, the baby can become infected with the herpes virus during birth. As a result the baby may suffer severe skin infection, damage to the nervous system, blindness, mental retardation, or death.

If you have ever had genital herpes or have had sexual contact with someone who has, tell your doctor. He or she may want to schedule more frequent examinations and possible testing to diagnose herpes.

If there are signs of active infection when you are in labor, your doctor may plan for a cesarean birth. Cesarean birth reduces the chance that the baby will come in contact with the virus in the vagina, because delivery takes place through a surgical cut in the abdomen. When there are no herpes lesions, the baby can be delivered vaginally.

Human Papillomavirus

Human papillomavirus is a virus that causes genital warts (sometimes called condyloma). Warts in the genital area are easily passed from person to person during sexual intercourse and oral and anal sex.

Although some warts may disappear on their own, in most cases treatment is needed. Warts often can be successfully treated during pregnancy. If warts are extensive, though, it may be best to wait until after delivery to begin treatment. In any case, your doctor will want to watch your condition closely throughout your entire pregnancy.

Syphilis

Syphilis remains a dangerous sexually transmitted disease. If untreated, it often spreads throughout the body and can cause blindness, heart disease, nervous disorders, insanity, tumors, and death. Syphilis can be passed from a pregnant woman's bloodstream to her fetus, sometimes causing ***miscarriage*** or ***stillbirth.*** If the infant lives, it may be born with congenital syphilis. Infants with congenital syphilis may have problems involving the nervous system, skin, bones, liver, lungs, or spleen.

Syphilis can be very hard to detect in women. The sore of ***chancre*** that marks the site of infection may be in the vagina where it cannot be seen. For most heterosexual men, the chancre appears on the penis, but it may be any where around the genital area.

In its early stages, when a chancre is present, syphilis may be diagnosed by examining the fluid from the chancre. A blood test may or may not find the disease in the earliest stages. The chancre will disappear even without treatment, but the disease remains. After the chancre has disappeared, the only sure method for diagnosing syphilis is a blood test.

Treating an infected pregnant woman will halt further damage to her fetus, but it will not reverse any harm already done. If treatment is completed during the first 3–4 months of pregnancy, it is very unlikely that the infant will suffer any long-term damage. Treating an infected infant after birth will usually prevent further damage but will probably not reverse any damage already done.

HIV Infection and AIDS

Human immune deficiency virus (HIV) infection and acquired immune deficiency syndrome (AIDS), the disease caused by HIV, are growing threats to women. Once in the bloodstream, HIV invades and destroys cells of the immune system, the body's natural defense against disease, leaving it open to harmful infections that can cause death. When a person infected with HIV comes down with one of these serious infections, he or she is said to have AIDS. Once established, the infection persists for life and is nearly always fatal. It may take more than 5 years for symptoms to appear; meanwhile, the virus can spread, both to sexual partners and to a fetus.

The virus is passed from person to person through body fluids: blood, semen (a mixture of sperm and fluid that a man releases during orgasm), and possibly vaginal fluid. The most common ways these fluids are exchanged are through contact with infected blood during intravenous drug use, sexual contact, and to a fetus from its infected mother's blood.

About one-third of the time, the virus is passed to the fetus during pregnancy. Most infected babies die within 3 years after birth. Because the virus can be passed across the *placenta* before birth, it makes no difference whether the baby is born trough the vagina or by cesarean delivery—infection may already have occurred. A mother who is breast-feeding may infect her infant after birth because the AIDS virus is present in breast milk. This means that even if a woman remains free of infection during her pregnancy, she could still pass the virus on to her newborn through her breast milk if she were to become infected shortly after delivery.

If you think that you may have been exposed to the AIDS virus. It is important to talk with your doctor about being tested. Research is ongoing, and it may be possible for the condition to be treated.

A test called the enzyme-linked immunosorbent assay (ELISA) is used to detect HIV. It will show whether your blood contains HIV *antibodies*—a sign that you have been infected. Positive result are then confirmed by Western blot, another test used as a double check. If both tests are positive, you are considered to be infected. A positive test does not mean that you have AIDS; it means that you have been infected with HIV and that you run a high risk of getting AIDS and passing it on to others. About 1 time in 20,000, the tests will give a false-positive result. A false-positive result means that the test indicates that you have been infected when you haven't been.

There are other factors that can cause less-than-accurate test results. After exposure to the virus, several weeks to several months are usually required before enough antibodies show up in the blood to produce a positive test result. This means that if you were exposed to the virus only a week before being tested, the test would show a negative result. A negative test can't tell you whether you are now infected; it only indicates that you didn't have antibodies when the test was done. A negative test also doesn't mean that you are immune to AIDS. You still need to protect yourself from infection.

You are at risk of being infected with HIV and getting AIDS if you:

- Use intravenous drugs
- Have sex with someone who has multiple partners, uses intravenous drugs, or is bisexual
- Had a blood transfusion before 1983

To protect yourself, your children, and others, you should change any risk-taking behavior and be tested for the presence of antibodies to the virus in your blood.

Medical Conditions

Some women have medical conditions, such as diabetes (high blood sugar), hypertension (highblood pressure), or cardiovascular (circulatory) problems that will call for special care during pregnancy. These medical problems are more easily managed if they are well under control *before* you become pregnant. This is another reason why talking to your doctor about your pregnancy plans in a good idea. The effects of these conditions during pregnancy are discussed in.

Pregnancy at 35 and Older

If you are in your mid-30s or older and are planning to have a baby, you're not alone. The trend toward delaying parenthood is a growing one. More and more couples are starting their families later in life. In the past decade, the rate at which women in their 30s had their first child almost doubled.

Most women who have children in their 30s or 40s have uncomplicated pregnancies and bear healthy children. Women who want to delay parenthood—or to continue to bear children in their 30s—often have concerns about their ability to become pregnant, the effects on their health, and the health of their baby. Some of these concerns are valid, but others are not. In general, women retain their good health and their ability to have healthy children into their 40s, although becoming pregnant may be more difficult.

Women age physically over time, not all at once. The potential for problems during pregnancy and childbirth does increase slightly each year beyond a woman's early 30s but there is no age at which there is a sudden dramatic change.

The risk of infant death within the first year of life is almost the same for babies born to mothers 25–19 years of age and to mothers 30–34 years of age. The risk increases slightly in women who have their first babies when they are 35–39, and more significantly once a woman reaches her 40s.

A woman's fertility gradually declines as she reaches her mid- 30s. One reason for this is that a woman ovulates—releases an egg for fertilization—less often as she ages. The number of eggs available for fertilization decreases with age, so you may not be ovulating every month, even though you have a menstrual period. You may spend several extra months trying to conceive before becoming pregnant. This wait can be trying if you are eager to become pregnant.

The likelihood of birth defects increases with age, but it remains low well into a woman's 30s. Women 35 and older are usually tested for genetic disorders such as Down syndrome, a disease that is linked to mental retardation and other medical problems. (Down syndrome used to be called mongolism, but this term is no longer used).

Any of these factors could be a risk, but they do not necessarily mean that you won't have a normal, healthy baby. They do require that you be informed about potential problems and discuss your plans with your doctor to ensure that you get the proper medical attention that any special concerns require.

Questions to Consider...

- should I gain or lose weight before pregnancy?
- Do I have any special dietary needs?
- Does my use of alcohol, tobacco, or drugs interfere with my chance of having a healthy pregnancy?
- Could any of the over-the-counter medications I'm taking be harmful to my baby?
- Should I start an exercise program? Cam I continue my present exercise program?
- Does my work expose me to things that could be harmful during pregnancy?
- Do I need to be vaccinated for any infectious diseases before I try to conceive?
- Should I be tested for any sexually transmitted diseases?

33

How Reproduction Occurs

A general understanding of the reproductive process, particularly fertilization and ovulation, will help as you prepare for pregnancy. Knowing how your body works will help you identify the time in your menstrual cycle when you are most fertile.

The Menstrual Cycle

A woman's fertility revolves around her menstrual cycle. Each month her ovaries produce an egg. The uterus is prepared for pregnancy by development of a thick lining in which the egg will grow if it is fertilized. If the egg isn't fertilized, the lining is shed during the menstrual period and the cycle begins again.

The changes that take place in the menstrual cycle are caused by hormones—substances normally produced by the body to control certain functions:

- **Follicle-stimulating hormone (FSH)** and **luteinizing hormone (LH)** are produced by the **pituitary gland** (a small organ located at the base of the brain) and cause eggs to mature and be released.
- **Estrogen** and **progesterone** are produced by the ovaries and prepare the lining of the uterus to nourish a fertilized egg.

Human chorionic gonadotropin (hCG) is produced by cells that eventually form the **placenta** once the fertilized egg has developed and attached to the uterine wall.

Days 1–5 of the menstrual cycle are called menstruation, during which the endometrium (lining of the uterus) breaks down and is shed through the vagina during your monthly menstrual period. This shedding is triggered by a drop in the levels of the hormones estrogen and progesterone, which occurs when an egg is not fertilized.

The drop in estrogen and progesterone signals the pituitary to send a surge of the hormone FSH to the ovaries. During days 1–13 of the menstrual cycle, FSH stimulates follicles in the ovaries to produce estrogen. Follicles are structures that produce the egg inside the ovary. Each month one follicle is the source of the egg for that cycle. The estrogen made by the follicle causes the endometrium to begin to thicken and develop. Cervical mucus becomes thinner and clearer during this phase.

Ovulation—the release of an egg from one of the ovaries—occurs on day 14 in the average 28-day cycle. The increased amount of estrogen produced by the follicles, in addition to stimulating the endometrium, also causes an increase in LH, which in turn triggers the follicle to release the egg. Once the egg is released, it can be fertilized for 12–24 hours.

After ovulation, the follicle is changed into the corpus luteum. During the second half of the cycle, the corpus luteum produces progesterone, which causes further thickening of the lining of the uterus.

When fertilization does not occur, estrogen and progesterone production drops sharply. This drop triggers the endometrium to shed, making the beginning of another menstrual cycle.

The average menstrual cycle lasts 28 days but may range from 23–35 days. The time frames given here for the various phases of the menstrual cycle are only averages. Your own cycle will probably vary somewhat from month to month. It's a good idea to keep a diary of your menstrual cycle so you will know what is normal for you.

If fertilization does occur, the developing placenta, which nourishes the fetus in the uterus, produces the hormone hCG. This is the hormone measured in pregnancy tests. During the early stages of pregnancy, hCG stimulates the follicle that has released the egg (the corpus luteum) to produce estrogen and progesterone. The increase in estrogen and progesterone that occurs during pregnancy prevents ovulation and menstruation during pregnancy.

Detecting Ovulation

Women who wish to plan when they become pregnant can do so by timing intercourse near the time they ovulate. There are several ways to detect ovulation. One way is by monitoring your basal body temperature. A woman using this method takes her temperature every morning before getting out of bed and records it on a graph. Most women have a slight but detectable rise in their normal body temperature after ovulation. This method is useful in showing a pattern you can use to predict when you will ovulate in future cycles. It cannot be used to predict ovulation in the month in which the temperature is recorded, because your temperature pattern is not complete until the month is over, and because you temperature does not begin to go up until ovulation has already occurred.

Another way to detect ovulation is by observing changes in the amount and makeup of the fluid, called cervical mucus, that normally is released from the vagina. Women who use this method learn to recognize the changes that occur in cervical mucus around the time of ovulation. The fertile period starts with the first signs of mucus and continues through the peak day.

Kits that will help detect ovulation can be purchased in a drugstore without a prescription. These kits contain chemicals that show the LH surge that comes just before ovulation. They must be used exactly according to instruction.

Fertilization

About every 28 days an egg is released from one of the ovaries into the nearby Fallopian tube. Once the egg is in the tube, it moves slowly toward the uterus. If a man's sperm does not fertilize the egg while it is in the tube, the egg continues down the tube to the uterus and is absorbed by the body.

Sperm cells are made in a man's testes, located in the scrotal sac below the penis. When the sperm cells mature, they leave the testes through small tubes called the vas deferens. These tubes carry the sperm to a larger tube in the penis called the urethra. As sperm travel from the testes, they mix with fluid from the seminal vesicles and prostate gland (a gland that produces most of the fluid for ejaculation). This mixture of sperm and fluid is called semen. When the man ejaculates or climaxes during intercourse, semen travels through the urethra in the penis into the vagina. It is not necessary for a woman to climax to become pregnant.

Pregnancy can occur if you have sexual intercourse during or near the time of ovulation. When the man ejaculates, his sperm are released into the vagina. They then travel up through the cervix, into the uterus, and out into the fallopian tubes. If live sperm meet a ripe egg in one of the tubes, fertilization can occur. The ripe egg can survive only about 12–24 hours, but sperm normally can live 2–3 days or longer. The fertilized egg then moves through the tube into the uterus and becomes attached there to grow and develop.

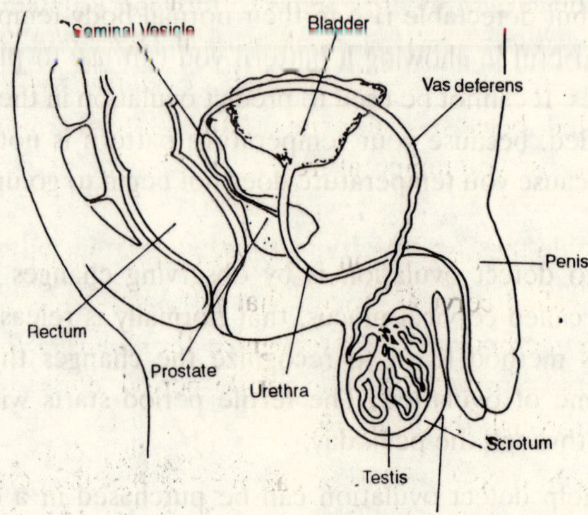

The male reproductive system

Infertility

Many couples who want a child face the problem of infertility—they have tried to conceive but have not been able to do so. Couples are considered infertile if they have not been able to conceive after 1 year of regular sexual intercourse without the use of any form of birth control. Infertility occurs in about 15% of all couples. If you don't get pregnant after trying for 6–12 months, you may wish to explore special tests and techniques.

The Infertility Evaluation

Couples who are infertile and want to conceive a child should think about having a complete infertility evaluation. Usually examinations for infertility begin with a medical history and general physical examination of the man and the woman. A medical history of the woman includes questions about any past illnesses, such as appendicitis or pelvic infections, that might have damaged her reproductive organs.

The couple will also be asked about their sexual relations to find out whether their infertility may be related to such factors as timing or frequency of intercourse. Often a couple may simply need more information on the sexual techniques that are most favorable to conception. Timing sexual intercourse to take place just before ovulation, for example, increases the chances of conception.

These initial examinations are then followed by more extensive testing of both the man and the woman to detect the exact cause of the infertility and to find out whether it can be treated. Depending on the cause of the infertility, alternatives are available.

Alternatives

If a woman is fertile and her partner is infertile, artificial insemination may be an option. For this procedure, semen is obtained from a donor who has been carefully screened for characteristics chosen by the couple. This screening also ensures that the donor does not have any serious diseases that could be transmitted to the woman. This semen, and the sperm it contains, is inseminated, or introduced, into the woman's vagina. At present, frozen instead of fresh semen is generally used.

If a woman is infertile because of blocked fallopian tubes, she may have surgery to open them. If surgery doesn't work, pregnancy may be possible with a procedure called **in vitro fertilization (IVF)**. It involves inducing ovulation with medications that cause multiple eggs to be produced. These eggs are removed from the ovary with the aid of a laparoscope or ultrasound. They are then fertilized with the man's sperm in a dish in the laboratory. The fertilized eggs are then transferred back into the mother's uterus through her vagina.

A variation of this technique is **gamete intrafallopian transfer (GIFT).** It is considered closer to normal fertilization than IVF because the egg and sperm are joined inside the woman's body instead of in a laboratory dish. After the egg and the sperm are obtained as for IVF, they are both put in the woman's fallopian tube, where the egg is fertilized.

These methods are new and may not be widely used in four area. They also involve special considerations that must be carefully weighed by a couple and their doctor. Such alternatives are not for everyone and usually are considered when other methods don't work.

34

A New Life Begins

After the sperm from the man enters and fertilizes the woman's egg in the fallopian tube, the fertilized egg becomes implanted in the wall of the uterus. The developing baby is called an embryo for the first 8 weeks after fertilization. After that it is known as a fetus. For all 40 weeks of pregnancy, the cells of the fetus grow and multiply at an incredible rate—from that first single cell that carries the "blueprint" for the baby's entire physical development to a completely formed individual weighing on the average about 7 pounds and measuring about 20 inches in length.

Early Signs of Pregnancy

The sign that most women associate with pregnancy is a missed menstrual period. But not all women have regular periods. Menstrual periods can be affected by stress or illnesses, so it is best to watch for a number of other signs:

- **Scanty menstrual period or spotting**
- **Breast tenderness**
- **Extreme tiredness**
- **Nausea**
- **Bloated sensation**

- Frequent urination

If you have one or more of these symptoms along with a missed period, you should consider that you may be pregnant, even if you have been using birth control.

Diagnosis of Pregnancy

It used to be necessary to wait until you missed two periods to have a pregnancy test. Today pregnancy can be confirmed about a week after you miss a period. During early pregnancy, the hormone called ***human chorionic gonadotropin (hCG),*** which is produced by the developing **placenta,** is present in the mother's urine and blood. You can take a urine sample to your doctor or to a clinic, or you can test it yourself with a home pregnancy test kit. If the test shows that you are pregnant, you should make an appointment with your doctor to confirm the pregnancy and begin prenatal care.

There are many home pregnancy test kits that you can buy without a prescription. All of the tests check for the presence of hCG in your urine. If your body has produced enough hCG, a chemical in the test kit will react with the hCG in different ways. In some, a ring forms in a liquid or a bead changes color.

In general, the tests require that you use a sample of the first urine you pass in the morning. It has the highest amount of hCG in it. Don't use the urine if it is cloudy or discolored. A small part of the urine will be added to a powder or liquid in the test kit. With some kits, the urine is mixed with the test solution and then left to sit for a certain amount of time. Other kits have more steps to follow, and you may need to time each of the steps accurately. The amount of time needed to get a result can vary, but often a result is available within an hour.

The test can easily give a wrong result if the directions are not followed. Be sure to follow the directions of the test exactly:

- Use only clean containers—never reuse the containers in the kit.
- Time the test for the exact number of minutes required.
- Leave the test in a place away from heat and where it will not be bumped.

A few medical conditions or some drugs can cause the test to turn out positive even if you aren't pregnant. A negative test may mean either that you are not pregnant or that you are pregnant but your body hasn't made enough hCG yet to be detected by the test. Many kits contain two complete tests so that you can test your urine again in a few days if the first test is negative.

Home pregnancy tests can be very accurate, but no test is 100% foolproof. False-negative results (showing you are not pregnant when you really are) can occur in a small number of cases. A blood test for pregnancy, performed in a laboratory, is more accurate. With home testing, a negative result—showing that you are not pregnant—should not be considered foolproof. The results of a home pregnancy test, whether positive or negative, should be confirmed by your doctor as soon as possible.

Growth and Development

During pregnancy the fetus grows in the mother's uterus. As described in Chapter 2, the uterus is located in the pelvic cavity between the bladder and the rectum. Almost as soon as pregnancy occurs, the lining of the uterus begins to thicken and its blood vessels enlarge in order to nourish the growing fetus. The uterus changes continually throughout pregnancy, expanding as the fetus grows.

The placenta begins to form and grow as soon as the fertilized egg attaches to the lining of the uterus. Also known as the afterbirth, the placenta is the channel through which oxygen, nutrients, drugs, hormones, and other substances pass from mother to fetus. In the opposite direction, waste products from the fetus cross through the placenta to the mother via the fetal vessels of the umbilical cord to be disposed of by her body.

The placenta starts as small sprouts growing from the wall of the fertilized egg. In these sprouts, called **chorionic villi,** fetal blood vessels form. The tips of the vessels enter the wall of the uterus and tap the mother's blood vessels. Although the maternal and fetal blood systems are in close contact, the two bloodstreams do not mix. The placenta is expelled from the uterus soon after birth.

Fetus

1st month:. By the end of the first month, the embryo has a head and a trunk. Features are beginning to form, and tiny structures called limb buds, which will grow into arms and legs, begin to appear. The heart also forms and begins to beat on the 25th day. At the end of this month, the embryo is about 1/2 inch long and weighs less than 1 ounce.

2nd month:. The early stages of the placenta, chorionic villi, are visible and working. All of the major body organs and systems are formed, although they are not completely developed. The heartbeat can be detected with special techniques. The first bone cells have appeared. Ears, ankles, and wrists are formed, and fingers and toes are developed. Eyelids form and grow but are sealed shut. At the end of the second month, the fetus is a little over 1 inch long but still weighs less than 1 ounce.

3rd month:. Fingers and toes of the fetus have soft nails. There are 20 buds for future teeth, and hair is beginning to appear on the fetus's head. Kidneys develop and secrete urine into the bladder. The initial stages of all organs can be recognized. From now on, the organs will mature and the fetus will gain weight. By the end of this month, the fetus is 4 inches long and weighs a traction over 1 ounce.

4th month:. The fetus moves, kicks, sleeps and wakes, swallows, can hear, and can pass urine. Eyebrows have formed, and there is a small amount of hair on the head. The skin is pink and transparent. The fetus is now 6–7 inches long and weighs about 5 ounces.

5th month:. The fetus has a real growth spurt. The internal organs are maturing. Fingernails have grown to the tips of the fingers. The fetus sleeps and wakes at regular intervals and is much more active, turning from side to side and sometimes moving head over heels. At the end of the month, the fetus is 8–12 inches long and weighs anywhere from 1/2 to 1 pound.

6th month:. The fetus in continuing its rapid growth, but its organ systems are still developing. The skin is wrinkled and red and covered with fine, soft hair. At the end of the sixth month, the fetus will be 11–14 inches long and weigh about 1 to 1 1/2 pounds. But because it is still so small and its lungs are not fully developed, it usually cannot live outside the mother without very specialized care.

7th month:. This is another rapid growth period for the fetus. It exercises by kicking and stretching. It sucks its thumb and opens and closed its eyes. Calcium is being stored, and fetal bones are hardening. The fetus now has a better chance of survival if it is born early. It is gaining weight—now weighing about 3 pounds—and is about 15 inches long.

8th month:. The fetus continues to grow in size and weight. It is too big to move around much, but its kicks are felt much more strongly, and the shape of a small heel or elbow may be visible to you through your abdomen. The bones of the head are soft and flexible. It is now about 18 inches long and weighs about 5 pounds.

9th month:. The fetus is now gaining about 1/2 pound per week. The bones of its head are soft and flexible for delivery. It is getting ready for birth and usually settles into a favorable position. It is curled up with its knees against its nose and its thighs tight against its torso, resting lower in the abdomen. At 40 weeks, it will be full term and weigh 6–9 pounds. Your baby should arrive anywhere from 37–42 weeks of pregnancy.

MOTHER

1st month:. You may not notice anything different, but your body is going through many changes. The lining of the uterus is thickening. The hormones **progesterone** and

estrogen are being produced in increasing quantities. Perhaps you have not had a period (a condition called **amenorrhea**), or this month's period was very different from normal ones (scanty bleeding or spotting). Your breasts are slightly enlarged and tender, and your nipples may have become more prominent. You probably need to urinate more often, but this will ease in midpregnancy.

2nd month:. The total volume of blood in your body increases to accommodate the growing fetus. Your breasts are still tender. You may still be having some of the early discomforts of pregnancy (described in "Physical Changes",) as your body continues to adjust.

3rd month:. As you gain weight, your waistline begins to disappear. You may need to start looking for a larger bra and maternity clothes.

4th month:. Your abdomen begins to swell with the increase size of the fetus this month. Your nipples and the area around them start to darken. A line running from your navel to you pubic hair may darken (**linea nigra;**). Especially if you have dark hair and fair skin, the skin on your face may darken. This condition is called **chloasma** and can be brought on or worsened by being in the sun. The next few months are usually some of the easiest in pregnancy, because most of the early discomforts have disappeared. Sometimes from the end of this month on, you may begin to feel the movement of the fetus. This is called **quickening** and feels like a fluttering of wings or like small bubbles. Let your doctor know when you first feel this, because it helps to establish or confirm your due date.

5th month:.This month your uterus has expanded to reach the height of your navel, and the skin of the abdomen stretches. If you have not already, you will begin to feel the fetal movements.

6th month:. This is your period of greatest weight gain. You may feel the fetus kicking. You may also experience a stitch-like pain at times down the side of your abdomen as the uterine muscle stretches.

7th month:. Increased growth of the fetus adds stress to your system, causing some discomfort. The breasts and uterus continue to increase in size. For some women, stretch marks may appear on the abdomen and breasts, and you may feel **B raxton-Hicks contractions,** false labor pains.

8th month:. Stronger contractions may be felt this month, and you may notice a leakage of **colostrum,** a fluid secreted from you breasts at the beginning of milk production. Aches and pains due to increased weight may now occur more frequently. Your uterus has grown so that the top part lies just under your diaphragm.

9th month:. You may now notice your navel protruding and shortness of breath. Toward the end of this month, when the baby drops into a lower position, you may be able to breathe easier and may have an increased need to urinate. Your cervix will soften, and contractions will increase. Colostrum leakage may be increasing. Discomforts caused by the pressure and weight of the fetus are common, and you often need to rest during the day. Your ankles may swell some at the end of the day.

The growth and development of a fetus has a dramatic effect on a pregnant woman. Although most women experience some of the same physical changes, other changes may be unique to each woman. No two pregnancies are alike. Even for the same woman, a second or third pregnancy may be very different from the first. Understanding the changes that take place in your body and in the growing fetus during pregnancy will help you prepare for the weeks and months to come. Pregnancy usually lasts 280 days, 40 weeks, or about 9 calendar months (or approximately 4 1/2 weeks each) from the beginning of a woman's last normal menstrual period.

Questions to Consider

- Did I perform my home pregnancy test correctly?
- Are my early signs of pregnancy normal?
- Now that I'm pregnant, how do I start a program of prenatal care?

35

Decisions, Decisions

Pregnant women have many options and choices. They range from how to prepare for childbirth to where you want the baby to be delivered and by whom. These important decisions will affect how comfortable you will be with your care. Thinking now about some of the decisions and working through them with your partner and your doctor will help your feel more confident and in control as you approach the birth of your baby. Knowing in advance where and by whom your baby will be delivered, preparing for the birth with childbirth classes, and exploring your options regarding breastfeeding and other aspects of your care will help your make decisions later.

Choosing a Doctor

Choosing who will care for you during your pregnancy and delivery may be one of your first decisions. Ideally, you have already chosen your doctor before pregnancy and have had a chance to discuss preconception issues. Some women decide on a hospital where they would like to deliver their baby and ask for a referral to a doctor who practices there.

Babies can be delivered by certified nurse-midwives, doctors in family practice, or obstetrician—gynecologists. Certified nurse—midwives are registered nurses specially educated to provide health care to women and their babies from early pregnancy through labor, delivery, and the period after birth. In most states, nurse—midwives must practice with a doctor. They refer patients to a doctor if problems occur. Doctors in family practice provide general care for most conditions, including pregnancy.

Obstetrician—gynecologists are doctors who specialize in the care of women. Most have gone through a 4-year course of specialized training called residency, after graduating from medical school, and have been certified by the American Board of Obstetrics and Gynecology. To be certified, a physician must complete a residency, and them pass a written and oral examination to show that he or she has obtained the special knowledge and skills required for the medical and surgical care of the female reproductive system and related disorders.

If an obstetrician—gynecologist is certified, he or she is eligible to become a Fellow in the American College of Obstetricians and Gynecologists (ACOG), the organization that represents the specialty on both a national and a local level in women's health care issues. ACOG offers a wide variety of continuing medical education programs to help physicians stay current with the latest scientific and clinical practice advances. The initials FACOG behind a doctor's name signify that he or she is a Fellow who specializes in women's health care. A Junior Fellow of ACOG who is in practice has completed a residency program and is preparing to undergo final certification as a specialist in obstetrics and gynecology.

Board-certified obstetricians may become further specialized. One of these subspecialty areas is maternal—fetal medicine. These doctors have additional special training and experience in caring for women whose pregnancies are complicated by medical or obstetric problems. These specialists usually se patients by referral from another doctor.

Many women like to visit doctors and interview them before making a final decision. Feel free to raise questions about other areas of concern to you or your partner. A number of points could affect your choice of a doctor:

- Is the doctor's practice convenient to your home or work?
- Where does the doctor have hospital privileges?
- How do you obtain emergency care outside normal office hours?
- Do you have any problems that may require special care?
- What are the doctor's fees, and how are they covered by your medical insurance plan, if you have one? If you need advice on insurance or a payment plan, the doctor's staff may be able to help.
- Does your insurance plan limit your choice to certain physicians?
- What is the doctor's attitude about questions of concern to you, such as breast-feeding, pain relief, presence of fathers in labor and delivery rooms, and use of birthing rooms?

Another factor to consider is whether the doctor is in a group, collaborative, or solo practice. In a group practice, constant coverage is provided by two or more doctors. You may have a primary doctor and receive care from the others on occasion. It is possible that one of the other members may deliver you baby. This also holds true for collaborative practice, in which a doctor and a nurse or certified nurse-midwife work as a team to provide care before, during, and after pregnancy. With a solo practice, one doctor provides complete care for all of his or her patients. In the event of illness or vacation, coverage is provided by another doctor, whom you meet in advance.

Both types of practices have advantages and disadvantages. The solo practice allows you to see the same doctor each time, but could involve interruptions, such as canceled appointments when babies arrive unexpectedly, as they often do. The group and collaborative practices have the efficiency of shared resources, but you will receive care from more than one care provider.

The Health Care Team

Many doctors coordinate a team of health care professionals to provide various types of care based on a woman's special needs during pregnancy. The team is made up of persons who will assist your doctor, as well as those who may serve as consultants. The following members may be on the health care team:

- Nurses, who assist obstetricians by providing information needed to diagnose medical conditions, patient education, counseling, and advice on pregnancy nutrition and care
- Childbirth educators, who teach prospective parents about conception, pregnancy, childbirth, and family life
- Certified nurse—midwives, nurses who are specially trained to provide care to women during pregnancy and birth
- Labor and delivery nurses, who help the doctor care for patients in labor and who provide immediate care for babies after birth
- Postpartum nurses, who help care for the mother after birth
- Neonatal nurses, who help care for the newborn
- Dietician or nutritionist, who provides advice and guidance on diet and nutrition and any special needs
- Social workers, who can provide counseling and information about community services for families
- Residents, who are doctors in training at a teaching hospital

During your pregnancy and delivery, your doctor may consult other specialists, who then become a part of the health care team:

- Maternal—fetal medicine subspecialist, to give advice if complications or problems arise
- Geneticist, to detect or manage any inherited disorders or provide counseling on whether such a risk exists
- Neonatologist or pediatrician, to provide special care for the newborn
- Anesthesiologist (a specially trained doctor) to give anesthesia

The health care team can aid your doctor in gathering important information about your pregnancy. This information is used to determine how best to manage your prenatal care and to assess special needs during labor and delivery.

The Setting

The areas for labor and delivery vary from one hospital to another. Your doctor will be able to give you information about the potions available. Many hospitals have responded to the desires of parents-to-be by offering birthing rooms where the family can participate. These rooms may be located in the hospital or nearby. Birthing rooms share the specialized staff and services of a more traditional labor and delivery suite, which may be needed if a problem occurs. They provide a comfortable setting for labor, delivery, and, usually, postpartum recovery. Some allow the mother to remain in the same room for the postpartum stay, so the entire birth process can take place in one room, often with family members present. These rooms are referred to as LDRs (labor/delivery/recovery) or LDRPs (labor/delivery/recovery/postpartum).

There are also freestanding alternative birthing centers that are not in or near a hospital. These centers may not offer all the services that may be needed if a emergency arises. Because of these limitations, a hospital is considered the safest place to give birth.

When selecting your care, you may wish to ask about policies regarding fathers or others in the delivery room. Most hospitals permit support persons to be present in both labor and delivery rooms. It is wise to know the hospital's policy in advance so you can plan accordingly.

Your Childbirth Partner

One of your early decisions will be selecting your childbirth partner to help you through pregnancy, labor, and delivery. Support by a partner from the beginning can ease a woman's pregnancy and help the course of labor and delivery go more smoothly. This person may accompany you on prenatal care visits to your doctor and will attend childbirth preparation classes to assist you in breathing and relaxation exercises. During labor, your partner will take an active role as a coach, helping you carry out what you learned and practiced in childbirth class.

The father of the baby is usually, but not necessarily, the partner. If for some reason the father is not involved in the pregnancy, there are others who can give support and participate actively. A support person can be any family member or friend who will help you and be there for you.

The concept of family-centered care, now widely embraced in modern obstetric practice, focuses on the physical, social, and psychologic needs of the family unit, regardless of the members who may make up that unit. Family-centered care can extend to family members and loved ones who wish to take part in the process.

Childbirth Preparation

pain or discomfort is a natural part of childbirth for most women. Most pregnant women are concerned about how they will cope with labor and childbirth. It is difficult to know in advance how much pain or discomfort you will have during birth or how you will deal with it. You may find it helpful to learn how pain can be relieved with childbirth preparation techniques or drugs, or a combination of both.

Childbirth preparation is a means of coping with pain and reducing discomfort. The most common methods of preparation—Lamaze, Bradley, and Read—are based on the theory that much of the pain of childbirth is caused by fear and tension. Although there are differences in specific techniques, classes usually seek to relieve pain through the general principles of education, support, relaxation, paced breathing, focusing, and touch.

If you want further information about a particular method of childbirth preparation, ask your doctor to refer you to a childbirth educator. Your doctor can also discuss with you the other types of pain relief that are available.

Options

Certain decisions, such as those involving breast-feeding, circumcision, sterilization, and selecting an infant car safety seat for the trip home, won't be implemented until after delivery; but they should be thought about in advance. Other issues that may come up during pregnancy that would benefit from preplanning include work and travel considerations, discussed in Chapter ??.

Breast-Feeding

One of the most basic decisions you will have to make about the care of your infant is how to feed him or her—with breast milk or formula. During pregnancy, your body prepares to make milk whether or not you plan to breast-feed. Breast milk, including the **colostrum** that appears in the first 2–4 days, is designed by nature to nourish and protect newborns. Infants who are breast-fed have fewer feeding problems, tend to be less constipated, and have fewer infections and allergies.

Others may help you in your decision. Find out partner's feelings. Ask your doctor, nurse, or childbirth educator any questions you may have. Talk with women who know—some who have breast-fed their babies and others who have decided against it. Your best choice will be the one with which you feel most comfortable.

Circumcision

Parents-to-be often have many questions about circumcision. A man or boy who has not been circumcised has a layer of skin (the foreskin) that covers most of the sensitive end of the penis. Circumcision involves cutting away this skin at the end of the penis. When circumcision is requested by the parents, it is usually done before the baby leaves the hospital.

There is controversy about the need for circumcision. Although it is fairly common in the United States, it is much less common in most other parts of the world. Some parents choose to have their sons circumcised for religious or cultural reasons. There are no laws or hospital rules that require circumcision, however. It is an elective procedure and should be the parents' informed choice.

Sterilization

Couples who decide that they do not want any more children may consider sterilization of either the man or the woman. Almost half of the women who choose sterilization have it done postpartum. It is often performed within a day after delivery, while the woman is still in the hospital.

Because sterilization is permanent, it is a decision that requires careful thought by you and your partner. It is not a decision to make at times of stress or near the end of pregnancy. Therefore, it is appropriate to consider this option as early in pregnancy as possible in order to plan in advance.

If you want to limit the size of your family, you may wish to wait until the health of your newborn is assured before making the decision to be sterilized. For further details about sterilization and other forms of family planning,

Infant Safety Seat

Make plans now to bring your infant home in a special infant safety seat. Some states have passed laws requiring the use of infant seats under penalty of fine, and many hospitals will not allow the baby to be discharged without one. A plastic infant carrier is not a safety seat, even if a seat belt is placed around it. It can shatter in an accident. There are various models of infant car seats that are specially designed to protect babies and small children from harm should a crash occur. The seats can be rented or purchased. Check with your doctor, hospital, car dealer, baby stores, or local consumer safety council about purchase or rental.

Questions to Consider...

- Who are the members of my health care team?
- What options are available in my community in choosing a hospital?
- Where can I enroll in a childbirth preparation class?
- Where can I obtain further information on breast-feeding, circumcision, and sterilization?
- How do I select an infant safety seat?

36

Prenatal Care

A program of prenatal care allows your doctor to monitor your health and that of your fetus throughout pregnancy. Although most pregnancies proceed normally, every pregnancy poses some degree of risk. Assessing the risk on an ongoing basis is a central part of prenatal care. At each visit, your doctor will examine you and chart the course of your pregnancy. New techniques provide exciting opportunities to study the fetus. Some of these techniques can help alert your doctor to potential problems.

Even if you previously had a problem-free pregnancy, you should still see your doctor early. No two pregnancies are alike, and complications can arise without warning. Some women who think they are pregnant may delay prenantal care because they are uncertain about continuing the pregnancy. Seeing your doctor can give you the information you may need to make this decision. Your doctor can provide referrals to other counselors, should you need such services in deciding how to manage your pregnancy.

Prenatal care is not just medical care. It also includes childbirth education, counseling, and support of the family. Your doctor can direct you to these services, and you can do your part by participating actively in them.

Regular visits to your doctor are central to your prenatal care. Your first prenatal visit will be longer and more involved than other visits. It will include a history of your health, laboratory tests, a physical examination, and confirmation of the estimated date of delivery—your due date. A schedule will then be set up for subsequent visits and any special tests or instructions you may need. Throughout the process, you should discuss all facets of care with your doctor, and you should feel free to raise questions.

Informed Consent

The process by which you learn what a medical procedure, test, or treatment involves before you grant permission for it is called informed consent. The informed-consent process begins in your doctor's office with a discussion of what you might expect and covers most aspects of your care as described in this book. It is important that you understand this information. Don't be afraid to ask questions or to have your doctor go over anything that isn't clear to you. The physician will note in your record that treatment and risks have been explained to you, and he or she will document your treatment decisions.

As partners in your medical care, both you and your doctor have rights and responsibilities. You have the right to:

- Quality care without discrimination
- Privacy
- Knowledge of the professional status of your care providers and their fees
- Be advised of your diagnosis, treatment, options, and the expected outcome
- Be give an opportunity to be an informed participant
- Refuse treatment
- Participate or refuse to participate in research or any experimentation that affects your care or treatment

You have the responsibility to:

- Provide your doctor with accurate and complete health information
- Let your doctor know that you understand the medical procedures and what you are expected to do

If you do not follow your doctor's plan, or if you refuse treatment, you must accept responsibility for your actions. Your doctor has the right to stop treating you as long as you have time to find another physician. While you are in his or her care, your doctor is responsible for providing you with the best care available.

History

One of the first things you will be asked to provide is information about your health, your family's health, and any past pregnancies. This information can be very helpful in detecting future problems. You are the only one who can provide this information, so it is important that your answers be honest, complete, and accurate. The information is kept private. This information is obtained during preconception care. If it was not, you will be asked to provide specific information about yourself, the baby's father, and your close family.

The medical history covers your general health. This includes whether you are taking any medications, have any allergies, have any medical conditions, or have been exposed to infections. It also covers your menstrual history, including your last menstrual period, and use of contraception. Information about habits that may place you at risk for problems during pregnancy, such as use of alcohol, drugs, or cigarettes and exposure to harmful agents, should also be provided.

The history of past pregnancies includes details about all former pregnancies and focuses on problems that may recur: the baby's weight at birth, how long labor lasted, method of delivery, any complications, or preterm labor. You will be asked to provide information about pregnancies that you may not have carried to full term.

The family history provides information about any genetic disorders that may be inherited. If you had a previous child with an inherited disease, genetic counseling and further studies may be needed. Your ethnic origin and general life style will also be covered to determine whether there are any factors that might affect your health or that of your baby.

Physical Exam

Once your health history has been obtained, the next step is usually a physical exam. During the physical exam, your height, weight, and blood pressure will be measured, and other parts of your body will be checked:

- Ears, eyes, nose, and throat
- Breasts, heart, lungs, and abdomen
- Extremities
- Lymph nodes
- Thyroid
- Skin and teeth

Your reproductive organs—cervix, vagina, ovaries, fallopian tubes, and uterus—are checked during a pelvic exam. The initial pelvic exam in often more comprehensive than one done at any other time. Although it can be slightly uncomfortable, this exam is important because the doctor will be checking for changes in your cervix (opening of the uterus) and the size of the uterus.

Early in pregnancy, the size of the uterus corresponds to the length of gestation—the length of pregnancy—and is used as a guide to establishing your due date. Until 12 weeks of gestation, your entire uterus fits inside your pelvis. At midpregnancy (20 weeks of gestation), its top generally reaches the navel. At term, the uterus will be under your rib cage.

When is the Baby Due?

The average length of pregnancy is 280 days, or 40 weeks, from the first day of the last menstrual period. However, a normal full-term pregnancy can last anywhere between 37–42 weeks of gestation. Only about 5% of babies arrive on the exact due date, and most women deliver within 2 weeks before of after this date.

Estimated Date of Delivery

Based on the information obtained at your first visit, your doctor will calculate your due date, also called the estimated date of delivery, or EDD (also known as the estimated date of confinement, or EDC). The method used most often is based on conception occurring 14 days after the start of the last menstrual period. The approximate date may be figured out by taking the date your last period began, adding 7 days, and then counting back 3 months. For example, if the first day of your last period was May 5, and 7 days to get May 12, then count back 3 months—the estimated due date is February 12. Because it can be difficult to predict the exact date, your doctor may use more than one method:

- If the date of ovulation is known, it is the most reliable method of determining the age of the fetus.
- Throughout pregnancy, but especially early on, a clinical exam, which shows the size of the uterus, can provide useful information.
- Pregnant women usually first feel fetal movements, or **quickening,** by 16–20 weeks.
- in a normal pregnancy, fetal heart tones can usually be heard by the doctor using a special stethoscope by 18–20 weeks, or at 12 weeks by using a **Dopler** device, a form of **ultrasound** that converts sound waves into signals you can hear.
- In the first half of pregnancy, ultrasound can be used to estimate the age of a fetus within 7–10 days. Later in pregnancy, this method is not as accurate.

Calculating the due date on the basis of your menstrual period is non always exact. Menstrual cycles differ from one woman to another, and the pattern of menstrual cycles affects the due date. Also, women often have lapses of memory about their periods. You can help by recording your periods and sharing this information with your doctor.

The Importance of Accuracy

The accuracy of the due date is confirmed by checking the size of the uterus and the regularity, length, and character of the menstrual cycle, including changes in bleeding. If there is doubt about the EDD, ultrasound can be used to confirm or define the date. The due date is important because certain tests, such as **amniocentesis** or **alpha-fetoprotein** testing must be done at a specific time in pregnancy and interpreted according to the length of pregnancy in order to get accurate results. The due date is also used as a guide for gauging the growth of the fetus and the progress of your pregnancy—important if the doctor needs to induce labor. If your condition and that of the baby don't correspond with the due date, your doctor can be in a better position to take steps to detect and manage problems if he or she is assured of the accuracy of the due date.

Estimated Date of Delivery

While the average pregnancy is 280 days from the last menstrual period, it is normal to give birth anywhere from 37–42 weeks after your last period.

Routine Tests

Several laboratory tests will be done early in your prenatal care, and some will be repeated at different times during pregnancy:

- *Blood tests* to identify your blood type, Rh factor, and other antibodies; to check for anemia and sexually transmitted diseases; and to determine whether you have had German measles (rubella) or have been exposed to hepatitis
- *Urine tests* to provide information about levels of sugar and protein and to detect possible infections
- *Pap test* to check for cervical cancer

In addition to routine tests, other tests may also be suggested, depending on your history, family background, or race. Routine screening for diabetes is recommended for women over 29 years old because they are more likely to have the disease, as are women with hypertension, obesity, and other risk factors, regardless of age. Some doctors prefer to screen all women because to is hard to assign an exact age when the risk becomes significant.

The information obtained at your prenatal visits may lead your doctor to suggest further tests to check on the status of the fetus. Some genetic tests may be offered routinely, such as a test to screen for alpha-fetoprotein that detects ***neural tube defects*** such as ***spina bifida***. Others may be recommended, particularly if you have a greater-than-average chance of giving birth to an infant with a birth defect. These tests are discussed in "Genetic Tests."

Future Visits

After your first prenatal visit, the following visits are usually shorter. The time during these visits is generally used to find out how you are doing and how the baby is growing and to address and special concerns you may have. You and your doctor will work out the timing of these visits, depending on your risk factors. You may follow a schedule somewhat like this one:

From the first visit to 28 weeks	Monthly
From 28 – 36 weeks	Every 2 weeks
From 36 weeks to delivery (at about 40 weeks)	Weekly

Women with medical or obstetric problems require more attention, whereas women who have no apparent risk factors may need less. Your doctor will want to see you more often if you have a problem or the potential for developing one.

During these visits, your weight and blood pressure are checked, and a urine sample is taken for testing. Your abdomen is measured to check the growth and position of the fetus, and the fetal heartbeat is checked on each visit. Lab tests and pelvic exams may not be done each time but may be spaced throughout the rest of your visits. These findings, as well as the results of the initial history, physical exam, and tests, will be noted on your medical record.

Throughout your pregnancy, your doctor will give you advice and counseling on leading a healthy life style. You are encouraged to ask questions during your prenatal visits. You should also make a note of any unusual signs or symptoms that may appear between visits. The diary at the back of this book can be used as a handy way to chart the course of your pregnancy.

Special Tests

Depending on your history and the results of your routine tests, your doctor may recommend that you have more tests to check the growth and health of the fetus. Some tests, such as ultrasound, allow you and your doctor to see an image of the fetus while it is in your uterus. This can be especially helpful for determining whether your fetus has grown and developed as expected for its age. Other types of tests result in a sound or recording of the fetus's heartbeat. Techniques may be used in combination to create both a sound and an image to assess the well-being of the fetus.

These tests cannot cure a problem, but they can alert your doctor that you may require special care. Although these tests are not fail-proof and so cannot guarantee a healthy baby, they can offer reassurance and help detect potential problems.

Ultrasound

Ultrasound, which creates pictures of the baby from sound waves, is available today in almost every major hospital and in many doctors' offices. This new technology has become useful for the general health care of women, but it is especially valuable during pregnancy and childbirth.

Ultrasound is energy in the form of sound waves produced by a small crystal. The sound waves move at a frequency too high to be heard by the human ear. They are directed into a specific area of the body through a device called a ***transducer***. The transducer is moved across the skin surface, scanning the area. The sound waves bounce off tissues inside the body, like echoes. They are converted into sounds of the heartbeat of the fetus, or images of the internal organs and the fetus, that appear on a television-like screen. Real-time ultrasound, the type that is used most often, quickly combines still pictures one after another to show movement, somewhat like the individual frames that make a motion picture.

The doctor will decide with you whether to use ultrasound and how often it should be done to best suit your needs. Ultrasound is often used to aid the doctor in detecting a suspected problem or checking a condition that has been confirmed. It can provide information that other tests and procedures do not.

In a way, ultrasound serves as a limited physical examination of a fetus. It can provide valuable information about the fetus's health and well-being, such as:

- Age of the fetus
- Rate of growth of the fetus
- Placement of the ***placenta***
- Fetal position, movement, breathing, and heart rate
- Amount of ***amniotic fluid*** in the uterus
- Number of fetuses
- Some birth defects

To prepare for an ultrasound exam, wear clothes that allow you to expose your abdomen easily, such as a top and a skirt or slacks. Some hospitals may ask you to wear a hospital gown.

A full bladder may be needed for your exam. You may be asked to drink several glasses of water 1 hour before the exam and not to urinate until after the procedure. A full bladder serves as a landmark, helping the doctor locate the pelvic organs. It also allows clearer, more accurate pictures. With ultrasound, the only discomfort you feel is that of a full bladder.

A doctor or an ultrasound technologist, someone specially trained in performing ultrasound exams, will conduct the test. As you lie on the table with your abdomen exposed from the lower part of the ribs to the hips, mineral oil or a gel is applied to the surface of the abdomen to improve contact of the transducer with the skin surface. The transducer is then moved along the abdomen. The sound waves sent out from the transducer enter the body and are reflected back when they come into contact with the internal organs and the fetus. The transducer may also be inserted in the vagina to aid in viewing the pelvic organs.

Although the effects of ultrasound are still being studied, no harmful effects to either the mother or the baby have been found in over 20 years of use. The long-term risks of ultrasound, if any, are unknown, but there are many benefits.

Fetal Heart Rate Monitoring

Ultrasound can be used to listen to the fetus's heartbeat. Sound waves are transmitted via an instrument that is held against the mother's abdomen or attached there with belts. Monitoring the fetus's heart can help show how it is responding to labor and also can give some helpful information before labor.

There are two types of electronic fetal monitoring that your doctor may use during pregnancy to check on the fetus. The ***nonstress test*** measure the fetus's heart rate in response to its own movements. The ***contraction stress*** test measures the fetus's response to contractions.

Nonstress Test. Usually the fetal heart rate increases when the fetus moves. The nonstress the measures the response of the fetus's heart rate to each of its movements, as felt by the mother or noted by a doctor or nurse. The heart rate is noted on a paper recording. If the fetus does not move for a short time during the test (perhaps as long as 40 minutes), it may be because it is asleep. If this happens, your doctor may try waking the fetus by using a buzzer.

The nonstress test may be combined with ultrasound to give a ***biophysical profile.*** The biophysical profile is most often used for women who are at increased risk of having a complicated pregnancy because of a medical condition such as high blood pressure of diabetes. The biophysical profile examines the fetus's breathing movements, muscle tone, body movement, and the amount of amniotic fluid (the liquid surrounding the fetus inside the uterus). Each of these items is given a score, and the total is added. As with electronic fetal monitoring, the biophysical profile does not cause any harm to the fetus, so it can be repeated weekly, if necessary, to check on the progress of your pregnancy. Your doctor may use the score to decide whether you need special care or whether your baby should be delivered early.

Contraction Stress Test. The contraction stress test measures how the fetal heart rate reacts to the temporary decrease in blood flow to the placenta that occurs during a uterine contraction. A normal response to this test implies that the fetus is receiving enough oxygen at the moment. This does not necessarily predict whether the fetus will respond well to future stress or labor, however. An abnormal response indicates the need for further testing and possibly treatment.

This test is often used if the nonstress test shows no change in fetal heart rate in response to fetal movement. Mild contractions of the mother's uterus are brought on by giving a drug called ***oxytocin*** or having the mother stimulate her nipples. The fetus's heart rate in response to the contractions is the recorded.

Risk Factors

A pregnancy is considered to be at increased risk when a problem is more likely than usual to occur. Such a problem could be caused by a health condition that the mother had before she was pregnant, or it may arise during pregnancy or at delivery. The small number of women who have recognized risks account for a large number of the problems that occur. Not all complications of pregnancy can be predicted, however. About 20% of infants who are in poor health or who die are born to mothers who did not have any signs of risk during pregnancy.

Factors that can Complicate Your Pregnancy

Medical

- Hypertension
- Heart, kidney, lung, or liver diseases
- Infections—sexually transmitted diseases, urinary tract infections, or other viral or bacterial infections
- Diabetes

- Severe anemia
- Convulsive diseases, such as epilepsy

Obstetric

- Problems in past pregnancies
- Mother younger than 15 or older than 35 years old
- Previous birth defects
- Multiple gestation (eg, twins or triplets)
- Bleeding, especially during the second or third ***trimester***
- Pregnancy-induced high blood pressure ***(preeclampsia)***
- Abnormal fetal fetal heartbeat
- Intrauterine growth retardation or prematurity (fetus not developed adequately for age)

Life Style

- Smoking
- Drinking alcohol
- Taking drugs not prescribed by physician (either illegal or over-the-counter drugs)
- Poor nutrition, including inadequate weight gain
- Lack of prenatal care
- Multiple sexual partners

Because problems can arise at any time, risks will be assessed throughout the pregnancy. Regardless of when problems occur, they can threaten the health of the mother or that of the fetus, or both. For this reason, a woman with an increased risk of complications will require more intensive prenatal care.

Questions to Consider...

- Is there anything in my history I may have overlooked that could pose a problem in pregnancy?
- When is my due date?
- What are the dates of my future visits?
- Will I need any special tests?

37

Genetics

Genetics is the study of how traits are passed on from parents to a child. Many personal traits are inherited this way, such as height and eye color. Unfortunately, some diseases can be passed on in the same way. A condition that affects a fetus and is present at birth is called a ***congenital disorder***. Through counseling and testing, you may be able to learn whether your fetus is at risk for having certain genetic diseases and congenital disorders.

Genes and Chromosomes

Normally, each male sperm and each female egg contain 23 gene-carrying chromosomes, or one-half of the 46 found in all other cells in the body. When an egg is fertilized by a sperm, the 23 chromosomes from the mother's egg and the father's sperm join to form the 46 chromosomes of the fetus. One pair of the chromosomes—one each from the sperm and the egg—are the sex chromosomes. There are two types of sex chromosomes, designated by the letters X and Y. A normal sperm will carry either an X or a Y; a normal egg is always X. If the union of an egg and a sperm is an XY, the child will be male; if XX, female. A man's sex chromosome thus decides the sex of his child.

Each chromosome carries many genes. Genes are responsible for the traits a person inherits from his or her parents. Genes come in pairs. Each parent contributes one-half of each pair of chromosomes and, thus, half the genes. Although some traits

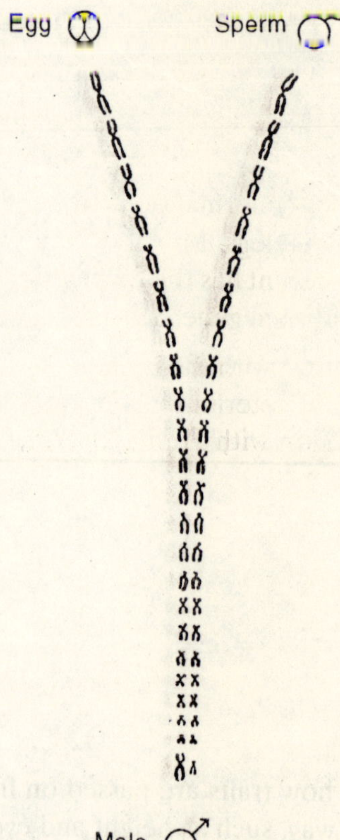

The fetus inherits 23 chromosomes each from its mother and father to make 23 pairs. The twenty-third pair determines the sex of the fetus: XX is female and XY is male.

are controlled by a single gene pair, others, including eye and hair color, are the result of many pairs of genes working together.

Genetic Disorders

Although most children in the United States are born healthy, about 2–3% of babies are born with some type of major congenital birth defect. Another 4–5% of babies are born with less serious problems, some barely noticeable or easily corrected. Although the cause of a birth defect is not always known, the cause of many genetic disorders is now well understood.

Dominant Gene Disorders

A dominant disorder needs only one gene from either parent to cause an effect on the child. The chances are 50–50 that any child (male or female) of this parent will inherit the gene. Following are some of the disorders that are passed on by a dominant gene:

- *Polydactyly* (having extra fingers or toes) is fairly common and can be corrected by surgery.
- *Achondroplasia* is a very rare abnormality of the skeleton in which a person has shorter-than-normal arms and legs. Most often it is the result of a new mutation, meaning that neither parent has the trait. When both parents are affected and each passes on the abnormal gene, the disorder is fatal.
- *Huntington disease* (a problem with the nervous system that causes uncontrollable movements and mental deterioration) usually affects people in their 30s or 40s. Each child of a person with Huntington disease has a 50% chance of having the disorder.

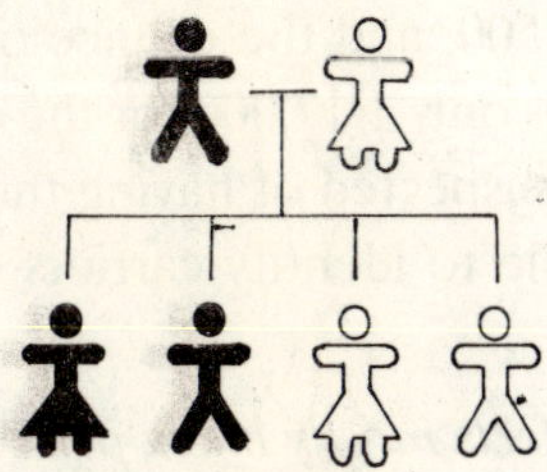

If one parent has a dominat gene disorder, there is a 50% chance that it will be passed to each child.

Recessive Gene Disorders

A genetic disorder can occur when a pair of the fetus's genes is made up of two abnormal recessive genes—one from each parent. Because there are so many genes within each cell, everyone carries a few abnormal recessive genes. Yet, in most people, no defect appears because the abnormal recessive gene is overruled by the normal gene.

In certain groups, it is more likely that the parents will both carry the same abnormal gene. For example, recessive disorders are more common in certain ethnic groups and in relationships between blood relatives. It is for this reason that marriages between first cousins and other near relatives are discouraged.

If both parents have a recessive disorder, all their children will have the disorder, too. If one parent has the disorder and the other does not (and isn't a carrier of the abnormal gene), all their children will be carriers, but none will have the disorder. Following are some common recessive disorders:

- *Cystic fibrosis* is the most common genetic disease among white persons of northern European descent. It causes the respiratory system to produce very

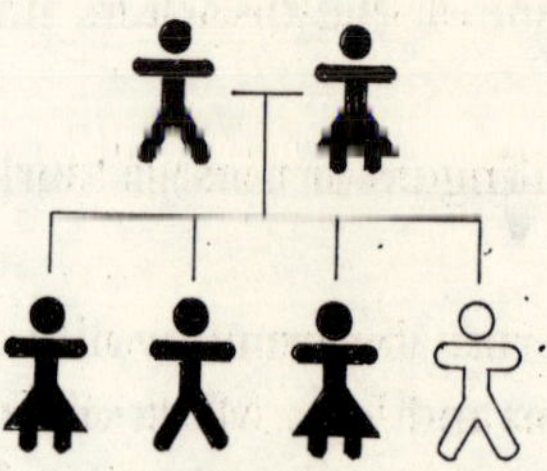

If both parents are carriers of a recessive disorder, there is a 25% chance that a male or female child will be affected and a 50% chance that a child (boy or girl) will be a carrier and not have the disorder.

thick mucus, clogging the lungs and causing lung disease. Most individuals with cystic fibrosis are infertile. Cystic fibrosis most often affects infants, children, and young adults. In the United States, the chance of a white person having the disease is about 1/2,500, and the chance of being a carrier is 1/25. For black Americans, the risk is only 1/17,000 for the disease and 1/50 for being a carrier. By testing a person suspected of having the cystic fibrosis gene and his or her relatives, it is possible to identify carriers of the gene and most fetuses who have the disease.

- *Sickle cell disease affects mostly black persons.* In the United States, about 1 in 625 blacks are affected, and about 1 in 10 are carriers. With sickle cell disease, the red blood cells take on a crescent, or "sickle" shape, rather than the normal "doughnut" shape. The abnormal, sickle-shaped red blood cells tend to get caught in the blood vessels, cutting off oxygen to tissues and causing pain. Because the body destroys these abnormal cells faster than it can make normal ones to replace them, anemia often occurs. Both carrier tests of the parents and prenatal tests of the fetus are available.
- *Tay-Sachs disease* is found mostly in persons whose families are of eastern European Jewish descent (Ashkenazi Jews). In this group, the disease occurs in 1 in 3,600 births. The chance of being a carrier is 1/30 for Ashkenazi Jews, but 1/300 for other persons. Symptoms first occur at about 6 months of age, progressively causing severe mental retardation, blindness, seizures, and death within a few years. Both tests for carriers and prenatal tests of the fetus are available.
- *Beta-thalassemia* causes anemia and is more likely to occur in persons of Mediterranean decent, such as Italians and Greeks. The risk for beta-thalassemia in these populations is between 1/2,500 and 1/800. The chance of being a carrier is about 1/25. Both carrier testing and prenatal testing of the fetus are available.

X-Linked Disorders

Some genetic disorders are determined by genes on the X chromosome and are thus referred to as X-linked or sex-linked. In most of these disorders, the abnormal gene is recessive. A woman can carry such a gene on one of her X chromosomes, yet not have the disorder because her normal gene on the other X chromosome prevents the disorder from being expressed. Because a male child will get one of his mother's X chromosomes, he may be affected. If the mother is a carrier for one of these X-linked disorders and the father is normal, there is a 50% chance that any given son will have the disorder and a 50% chance that any of their daughters will be a carrier. Very rarely, a daughter can inherit certain X-linked recessive disorders if, for example, her father and mother both have the disease.

Hemophilia is an X-linked disease. Persons with hemophilia lack a substance needed for blood clotting. Internal bleeding can be life-threatening to people with hemophilia, because they are very slow to stop bleeding. Hemophilia occurs in about 1 in 2,500 male babies. Testing a sample of blood will show whether an individual has hemophilia, and prenatal testing of the fetus is available.

Chromosomal Disorders

Genetic disorders may also be caused by problems with the fetus's chromosomes. Some of these are inherited, but most are caused by an error in the development of the egg or sperm. Having extra or missing chromosomes, or parts of chromosomes, usually causes serious medical problems. Most children born with chromosome disorders are mentally retarded in addition to having physical defects. The risk of having a child with a chromosomal abnormality increases with the age of the mother. The chance that a 35-year-old woman will have a child with any type of chromosomal abnormality is about 1 in 200; for a 40-year-old woman, the chance in about 1 in 60. Chorionic villus sampling or amniocentesis (described later) can identify fetuses with chromosomal disorders before birth.

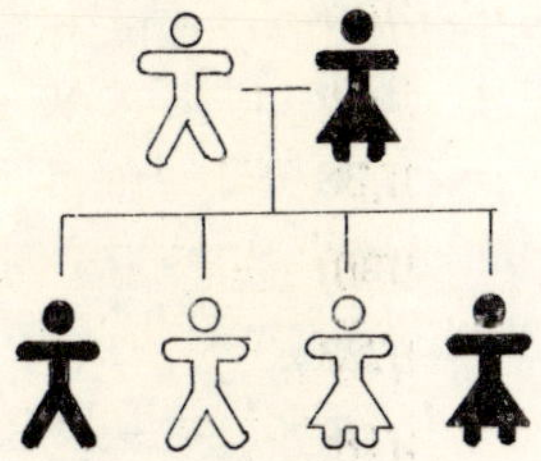

If a woman is a carrier of an X-linked (or sex-linked) disorder, there is a 50% chance that she will pass the disorder to her son and a 50% chance that her daughter will be a carrier.

Risk of Having a Baby with Chromosomal Disorders

Mother's Age	*Risk of Having a Live Baby with:*	
	Down Syndrome	*Any Chromosomal Disease*
20	1/1,667	1/526
21	1/1,667	1/526
22	1/1,429	1/500
23	1/1,429	1/500
24	1/1,250	1/476
25	1/1,,250	1/476
26	1/1,176	1/476
27	1/1,111	1/455
28	1/1,053	1/435
29	1/1,000	1/417
30	1/952	1/385
31	1/909	1/385
32	1/769	1/322
33	1/602	1/286
34	1/485	1/238
35	1/378	1/192
36	1/289	1/156
37	1/224	1/127
38	1/173	1/102
39	1/136	1/83
40	1/106	1/66
41	1/82	1/53
42	1/63	1/42
43	1/49	1/33
44	1/38	1/26
45	1/30	1/21
46	1/23	1/16
47	1/18	1/13
48	1/14	1/10
49	1/11	1/8

Of the disorders affecting one of the autosomal chromosomes, Down syndrome is the most common. Like other chromosomal disorders, the risk increases with the age of the mother: it is 1 in 1,667 live births for 20-year-old mothers, 1 in 378 live births for 35-year-old, and 1 in 106 live births for 40-year-olds. Affected children are mentally retarded and have a characteristic facial appearance. Persons with Down syndrome usually have three (celled trisomy) number 21 chromosomes instead of the normal two. Trisomy can also occur with other chromosomes: numbers 13 and 18, for example. These children are severely retarded and have many physical defects.

Other chromosomal disorders can occur when a person has too many or too few sex chromosomes. Men can have either an extra X chromosome or an extra Y chromosome. Males with Klinefelter syndrome have an extra X chromosome—that is, two X chromosomes and one Y chromosome. They have testicles that are smaller then normal and may be infertile; some are mentally retarded. Klinefelter syndrome affects about 1 in 800 men. Slightly less common is having one X chromosome and two Y chromosomes. Men with an extra Y chromosome may be taller than normal.

women can have just one X chromosome (Turner syndrome). Women with Turner syndrome tend to have puffiness of the hands and feet and webbing at the back of their necks. They may have incomplete development of their secondary sex characteristics, but early hormone treatment can help modify this. They are almost always infertile. The risk for Turner syndrome is about 1/3,000.

Multifactorial Disorders

Many disorders are thought to be somehow the result of multifactorial inheritance—a mix of genetic and environmental factors. The frequency of these disorders may vary in different parts of the world. some can be detected in pregnancy, but most cannot. A couple who has a child with a disorder of multifactorial inheritance usually has a 1–5% chance of having the disease affect future children. Two common multifactorial disorders are congenital heart defects and neural tube defects.

Congenital heart defects occur in about 1 in 125 infants. Although there are other causes of congenital heart defects, such as infection with rubella virus (German measles) or a specific chromosome problem, about 90% of the time these defects are the result of multifactorial inheritance. Congenital heart defects can sometimes be identified before birth by ***ultrasound***. In most cases, if parents have one child a with congenital heart defect, their chance of having another child with a heart defect is about 2–4%.

Neural tube defects occur when the tube enclosing the spinal cord does not close completely or form properly. In the very early stages of pregnancy, a long, narrow groove forms on the surface of the embryo, eventually deepening and then closing around itself to form a tubelike structure. It is from this neural tube that the spinal cord will develop, with the brain forming at one end. Only 1–2 pregnancies per 1,000 result in babies born with a neural tube defect.

The two major types of neural tube defects are ***anencephaly*** and ***spina bifida.*** Anencephaly occurs when the brain and head do not develop normally. Because the upper part of the brain is absent or underdeveloped, babies with this disorder are almost always ***stillborn*** or die shortly after birth.

Spina bifida has been called "open spine", because sometimes when the lower part of the neural tube doesn't close during embryo development, the spinal cord and nerve bundles are exposed outside the baby's body. This defect can be fatal, or it can result in serious long-term problems.

The other form of spina bifida, in which the defect is covered with skin, can also result in handicaps. However, they occur less often and are usually less severe than those associated with open spina bifida. With surgery and physical therapy, many children with a mild neural tube defect can lead relatively normal and productive lives.

The following disorders also can be passed on through multifactorial inheritance:

- *Clubfoot*—The affected foot is twisted at the ankle.
- *Cleft lip and palate*—A gap or space in the lip or a hole in the palate (roof of the mouth). When parents have already had a child with a cleft lip and palate, they have about a 4% chance of having another affected child. If they have had a child with cleft palate alone, they have a 2% chance of having another affected child.
- *Hip dislocations*—The ball and socket of the hip joint do not fit together well. This occurs more often in girls than in boys.

Counseling

Certain couples have a higher risk of having a baby with a birth defect. These include couples who have already had a child with a birth defect or who have a history of genetic disorders in their family. Women aged 35 and older are also at risk, as are couples of certain ethnic and racial backgrounds. If you are at increased risk of having a genetic disorder, genetic counseling is recommended. As a part of the counseling, you will be asked to recall family medical histories as far back as possible. This will help your doctor or a geneticist (someone who has special training in genetics) to determine your risk for various diseases. Certain tests also can show whether your fetus is affected.

The results of exams, tests, and histories will be explained, and the risk of a birth defect will be calculated. No test is 100% accurate, however. Your fetus may have a birth defect even if the test for it is negative or may be free of that defect even if the test is positive.

Less than 3% of all babies are born with a birth defect. Some defects are more likely to recur if you have already had one child with that defect.

The information you learn through genetic testing and counseling can help you make some important choices. If you or your partner is found to be a carrier of a genetic disorder, you will want to know what the risk is that the disorder may be passed on to any child you decide to have. Depending on the circumstances, you may choose to build your family by adoption. If the father is a carrier of a genetic disorder and the mother is not, you may want to consider artificial insemination. which is described in.

Risk of Genetic Disorders

Disorder	*Risk of Having a Fetus with the Disorder*	
	Overall	*With One Affected Child*
Dominant gene		
Polydactyly	1/300–1/100[1]	50%
Achondroplasia	1/23,000	50%
Huntington disease	1/15,000–1/5,000	50%
Recessive gene		
Cystic fibrosis	1/2,500[2]	25%
Sickle cell anemia	1/625[1]	25%
Tay–Sachs disease	1/3,,600[3]	25%
Beta-thalassemia	1/2,500–1/800[4]	25%
X-linked		
Hemophilia	1/2,500 men	50% for boy, 0% for girl
Chromosomal		
Down syndrome	1/800[5]	1–2%
Klinefelter syndrome	1/800 men	N/S[6]
Turner syndrome	1/3,000 women	N/S[6]
Multifactorial		
Congenital heart disease	1/125	2–4%
Neural tube defects	1–2/1,000	2–5%
Cleft lip/cleft palate	1/1,000–1/500	2–4%

Genetic Tests

Based on your personal medical history, your family medical history, and other factors, your doctor may offer certain special procedures of tests to detect genetic disorders. These tests are not cures, nor can they be expected to detect all potential problems. A specific test can be used to identify a specific problem, however, giving valuable information about the risk to your fetus.

In addition to the procedures described, there is a new method called percutaneous umbilical cord blood sampling (PUBS), in which a sample of the fetus's blood is checked for some diseases. This technique has risks, is very new, and may not be available in your area.

Alpha-Fetoprotein

Some tests are used to screen pregnant women for a disorder regardless of whether they have any risk factors. Measuring a chemical called ***alpha-fetoprotein(AFP)*** by a simple blood test can help identify women who might be carrying a fetus with a neural tube defect, a condition that often arises without warning. This test is called maternal serum AFP (or MSAFP) screening.

AFP is a protein produced by every growing fetus. Some of this protein is passed into the ***amniotic fluid*** that surrounds the developing fetus inside the mother's uterus. A smaller amount crosses the ***placenta*** (or afterbirth) into the.mother's blood. When the fetus has an open neural tube defect, large amounts of AFP leak into the amniotic fluid and then into the mother's blood. When the defect is covered by skin, however, the AFP is less likely to leak into the amniotic fluid. This type of neural tube defect is harder to detect by AFP testing or ultrasound. Low AFP levels have also been linked to a possible increased risk of Down syndrome.

For the MSAFP test, a small amount of blood is taken from the mother's arm. It is recommended that MSAFP testing be performed between 15–18 weeks of pregnancy. In order to interpret the MSAFP test properly, it is important to establish the age of the fetus as accurately as possible. Timing is also important for another reason: if the first test result are positive (higher or lower than would be expected at that point in pregnancy), enough time must remain in the pregnancy for further steps in the testing process.

If the result of the first blood test are negative, no further tests are needed. Yet this is no guarantee. Neural tube defects or Down syndrome may occur with negative test results. The AFP test can be a useful indicator. It will identify 90% of fetuses with anencephaly (lacking a brain) and 75% of those with spina bifida (having an opening in the back that exposes the spinal cord). It will identify about 25% of fetuses with Down syndrome in women under age 35.

For every 1,000 women tested, about 50 have an elevated AFP test. Of these 50, only 1–2 with higher-than-normal tests are carrying fetuses with a neural tube defect. Other possible causes for a positive test include incorrect dating of pregnancy, twins, or other conditions relating to high levels of AFP. Positive first test results, for whatever reason, mean that further testing is necessary. Those women whose test results are positive are offered further counseling and testing, which may include ultrasound and amniocentesis.

Amniocentesis

In ***amniocentesis,*** a sample of amniotic fluid is withdrawn through a needle. The amniotic fluid is then tested for certain genetic disorders. Amniocentesis is usually done at 14–18 weeks of pregnancy and can be performed on an outpatient basis, either in a hospital or in the doctor's office.

For the procedure, the patient is asked to lie down on an examining table, and her abdomen is uncovered. With the aid of ultrasound, a slender needle is carefully guided through the abdomen into the uterus and the amniotic sac. A small sample (about 1 ounce) of fluid is withdrawn through the needle (this fluid is replaced in a short time). This fluid is sent to a laboratory for testing. A number of fetal cells will be present in the amniotic fluid. The fetal cells in the fluid are grown in a special culture and then analyzed. The specific tests that are done will depend on your personal and family medical history.

Amniotic fluid is also tested for the level of alpha-fetoprotein as another means of detecting birth defects.

It can take about 2–4 weeks for enough fetal cells to grow so that a diagnosis can be made. These cells are prepared in such a way that their chromosomes can be studied under a microscope. The presence of an extra chromosome (as occurs in Down syndrome) or other chromosomal abnormalities can be diagnosed by such study. Because the sex of the fetus is also revealed by the test, amniocentesis may be used to help determine the risks of a sex- linked disorder.

Although complications from amniocentesis are uncommon, there is some risk involved. Occasional side effects include cramping, vaginal bleeding, and leaking of amniotic fluid after the procedure. Injury to the fetus is rare.

Miscarriage (loss of a pregnancy before the fetus is able to survive outside the uterus) occurs in about 3% of all pregnancies from 16 weeks of pregnancy onward, even if amniocentesis is not performed. With amniocentesis, the risk of miscarriage is increased up to about 0.5%.

Chorionic Villus Sampling

Chorionic villi (singular, villus) are microscopic, finger-like projections that make up the placenta. Villi come from the same fertilized egg as does the fetus and therefore reflect the fetal genetic makeup. In chorionic villus sampling (CVS), some of the chorionic villi are withdrawn through a needle that is inserted through the abdomen and into the edge of the placenta inside of the uterus. Villi can also be drawn through a catheter that is inserted through the vagina and cervix into the placenta. These cells are then grown in a special culture, and their genetic makeup, which is identical to that of the fetus, is analyzed.

In contrast to amniocentesis, which is performed in the second **trimester** of pregnancy, CVS can be performed during the first trimester, allowing for earlier detection of genetic defects. The results can be obtained more quickly—within about 10 days—allowing a diagnosis to be made, usually before the end of the first trimester.

As with amniocentesis, there are some risks with CVS. The most common complication is miscarriage. The risk of this happening is still fairly low, though—up to 1% higher than if CVS isn't done.

Amniotic Fluid

The fetus develops inside a sac formed by two membranes, the amnion and the chorion. Inside the sac, a liquid called amniotic fluid collects to support and protect the fetus. This watery environment in which the fetus grows is always changing: new amniotic fluid is being formed constantly, and some of the old is swallowed by the fetus.

Amniotic fluid begins forming during 4–5 weeks of pregnancy. At first it is composed almost entirely of fluid from the mother. As early as 11 weeks, the fetus's kidneys start to produce a weak urine. From midpregnancy onward, the fetus's urine is the main source of the fluid.

Amniotic fluid cushions the fetus, distributing evenly any shocks to the mother's abdomen. Because the fluid exerts pressure on the walls of the uterus, the fetus has room to grow. In a safe, temperature-controlled environment, the fetus can practice the movements it will need after birth. It can exercise its muscles by moving around, and as it breathes in and swallows the fluid it develops both a swallowing and a breathing mechanism. Amniotic fluid also discourages the growth of some kinds of bacteria, helping to protect the fetus from infection.

Abnormal Test Results

If one or more of your genetic tests has been positive, then the chance of your having a baby with a defect is increased. The facts and your feelings should be discussed with your partner, doctors, and counselors. This is often a difficult time for couples expecting a baby. Counseling can be very helpful in determining why your fetus is at risk for this disease and what options you have now and in the future.

If you are carrying a fetus with a genetic defect, you are faced with a difficult choice: You can choose either to end the pregnancy of to begin preparing for the birth of the child. This decision requires a great deal of thought, and often it may have to be made more quickly than you would like. Every couple has a different set of resources and values, so a decision that is right for one couple may not be right for another.

If you decide that the best course for you is to end the pregnancy in an abortion, it will most likely be done soon. The earlier the abortion is done, the simpler and safer it is for the woman.

Other couples elect to continue the pregnancy and have the baby. If you decide to have the baby, it is helpful to use the time remaining in the pregnancy to prepare yourself and your family. You may want to read about the condition your child may have or to join a support group. Along with your doctor and your family, you may start to plan the best possible care for your child beginning at birth. It may be difficult to predict how severely affected the child will be. Regardless of the decision you make, you may find counseling helpful in coming to terms with these issues.

Questions to Consider...

- What is the chance of my baby having a genetic disorder?
- Could my partner or I be a carrier of a genetic disorder?
- Should I have an alpha-fetoprotein test or amniocentesis?
- Should I have amniocentesis or CVS?

38

A Healthy Life Style

Many of the choices you make in your daily life affect your fetus. This is true of the things you do—exercise, rest, and work—as well as the things you don't do—expose your fetus to drugs, alcohol, cigarettes, or other risks. Some women may need to change their life style during pregnancy. This change not be easy, but your doctor and the health care team can give you information and support. Even better is the daily support of your family and friends, and especially your partner. Together, you can construct a healthy life style that will benefit you and your baby.

Exercise

Regular exercise during pregnancy can lead to a better appearance and posture, enhance your feeling of well-being, and lessen some of the discomforts of pregnancy, such as backache and tiredness. The goal of exercise during pregnancy should be to reach or keep a level of fitness that is safe.

What you can do in sports and exercise during pregnancy depends on your own health and, in part, on how active you were before you became pregnant. This is not a good time to take up a new, strenuous sport, but if you were active before your pregnancy, you should be able to continue, within reason. Caution should be the rule.

Here are some general guidelines for following a safe and healthy exercise program geared to the special needs of pregnancy:

- Regular exercise (at least three times per week) is better than spurts of heavy exercise followed by long periods of no activity.
- Brisk exercise should not be performed in hot, humid weather or when you have an illness with a fever, such as a cold or flu.
- Avoid jerky, bouncy, or high-impact motions. Activities that require jumping, jarring motions, or rapid changes in direction may cause pain. Exercise on a wooden floor or a tightly carpeted surface to reduce shock and provide a sure footing. Wear a good-fitting, supportive bra to help protect your breasts.
- Avoid deep knee bends, full sit-ups, double leg raises, and straightleg toe touches. During pregnancy, these exercises may injure the tissue that connect your leg and back joints.

Prenatal Exercises

There are a number of exercise programs designed especially for pregnant women. Your doctor can help you select exercises that are best for you.

Head and Shoulder Circles

Slowly moving your head and shoulders in circles can help relieve upper backache and tension in your head, neck, and shoulders.

- Stand or sit in a comfortable position.
- Inhale while slowly dropping your head toward your left shoulder and circling it to the back and on toward your right shoulder.
- Exhale while slowly letting your head circle to the front and around to your left shoulder again.
- Repeat several times.
- Inhale while slowly moving your right shoulder forward and then upward to form the top half of a circle.
- Exhale while slowly moving your shoulder to the back and then down to complete the circle.
- Repeat with your left shoulder.
- Do three to five repetitions.

Forward Bend

This exercise stretches and relaxes the muscles in your back to help relieve tension and fatigue.

- Stand with your feet about 12–18 inches apart and your knees slightly bent. (As you do this exercise, spread your legs, bend your knees, or do both, as needed for comfort. Don't try to keep your knees straight).
- Exhale and bend forward from the waist, letting your upper body slowly sag toward the floor, uncurling slowly.
- Inhale and slowly uncurl your back, one vertebra at a time, until you are once again standing up straight. (Do not try to keep your back straight or to rise quickly to a standing position, because you may become dizzy).

Arm Reaches

Stretching your side and upper body helps relieve upper backache. It is also helpful when you feel short of breath.

- Stand or sit in a comfortable position.
- Inhale as you raise your right arm above your head, reaching as high as you can. (Be sure to stretch from the waist, without letting your hip or foot rise).
- Exhale, bending your elbow and pulling your arm back down to your side.
- Repeat on your left side.
- Do three to five repetitions.

Pelvic Tilt

Tilting your pelvis back towards your spine can help strengthen your abdominal muscles and relieve backache. This exercise can be done in either a kneeling or standing position.

Standing

- Stand in a comfortable position.
- Inhale and relax.
- Exhale as you roll your hips and buttocks forward, as if trying to lift the fetus up toward your chest.
- Hold for a count of five.

- Inhale and relax.

Repeat three to five times, several times a day.

Kneeling

- Kneel on your hands and knees, with your back relaxed but not arched.
- Inhale and relax a moment.
- Exhale and pull your buttocks under and forward (you should feel your abdomen tighten and your back straighten at the waist).
- Hold for a count of five.
- Inhale and relax.

Side Leg Stretches

This exercise improves your circulation and tones and strengthens the muscles of your hips, buttocks, and thighs.

- Lie on your left side, with your knees, hips, and shoulders in a straight line Put your right hand on the floor in front of ycu, and use you left hand to support your head.
- Inhale and relax.
- Exhale while slowly raising your right leg as high as you can without bending your knee or body. Keep your foot flexed, with your right outside ankle bone facing up.
- Inhale while slowly lowering your leg.
- Repeat 10 times.
- Turn to your right side and repeat 10 times with your left leg.

Leg Stretches

Stretching your legs relieves tension in your hips and legs and helps relieve or prevent leg cramps.

- Sit on the floor with your right leg stretched out toward the side, your foot flexed, and your left leg folded in.
- Facing forward, lean your upper body to the right side, so that your right ear is directly over your right leg. At the same time, lift your left hand over your head, so that it is directly over your left ear.

- Using your right hand, grasp your right foot—or you ankle or calf if your cannot reach your foot comfortably.
- Hold this position for a count of 10.
- Relax and release the stretch.
- Repeat on the left side.
- Do three times (as you feel more comfortable with this exercise, try to hold the stretch longer).

You can change this exercise two different ways for more variety:

1. Instead of raising your leg all the way up, raise it only halfway and make small circles with it. Make 10 clockwise circles and then 10 counterclockwise circles.

2. Instead of keeping your upper leg straight, bend your knee so that your upper thigh is at a right angle to your body. Keeping your knee bent, do the side raises, making sure that your knee faces forward and your outer ankle bone faces upward.

- Avoid exercises that require lying with your back on the floor for more than a few minutes after 20 weeks of pregnancy.
- Always begin with a 5-minute period of slow walking or stationary cycling with low resistance to warm up your muscles. Intense exercise should not last longer than 15 minutes.
- Heavy exercise should be followed by a 5–10-minute period of gradually slower activity that ends with gentle stretching in place. To reduce the risk of injuring the tissue connecting your joints, do not stretch as far as you possibly can.
- The extra weight you are carrying will make you work harder as you exercise at a slower pace. Measure your heart rate at peak times of activity. Do not exceed your target heart rate and limits established with your doctor's advice.
- Get up slowly and gradually from the floor to avoid dizziness or fainting. Once you are standing, walk in place for a brief period.
- Drink water often before and after exercise to prevent dehydration (lack of enough water for the body's needs). Take a break in your workout to drink more water if needed.
- Women who did not regularly exercise before becoming pregnant should begin with physical activity of very low intensity and move to higher levels of activity very gradually.
- Stop your activity and consult your doctor if any unusual symptoms appear, such as the following:
  - Pain

- Bleeding
- Dizziness
- Shortness of breath
- Palpitations (irregular heartbeat)
- Faintness
- *Tachycardia* (rapid heartbeat)
- Back pain
- Pubic pain
- Difficulty walking

Almost any form of exercise is safe if it is done in moderation. Some exercises offer aerobic conditioning of the heart and lungs: others relieve stress and tone muscles. Pregnancy causes many changes in your body. Some of which have an effect on your ability to exercise.

- *Walking* is always good exercise. If you were not active before you became pregnant, walking is a good way to begin an exercise program.
- *Swimming* can be continued if you were used to swimming before pregnancy. Swimming is excellent for your body because it uses many different muscles while the water supports your weight. However, it is best not to dive in the later months of pregnancy. Scuba diving is not recommended during pregnancy.
- *Jogging* can be done in moderation if you were used to jogging before you became pregnant. Avoid becoming overheated, stop if you are feeling uncomfortable or unusually tired, and drink water to replace what you lose through sweating.
- *Tennis* is generally safe if you were used to playing tennis before pregnancy, but be aware of your change in balance and how it affects rapid movements.
- *Golf and bowling* are fine for recreation but don't really strengthen the heart and lungs. With either of these sports, you may have to adjust to your change of balance.
- *Snow skiing, water skiing, and surfing* pose some risk. You can hit the ground or water with great force, and taking a fall at such fast speeds could harm you or your fetus. Before you decide to participate, you should talk with you doctor.

Most couples can continue to have intercourse until shortly before the baby is born. sometimes couples are afraid that the act of intercourse will harm the fetus and cause a ***miscarriage***—this is not true. The fetus is well cushioned by the ***amniotic fluid*** surrounding it.

For your comfort, you and your partner may want to try different sexual positions. For example, intercourse with the man and woman on their sides causes less pressure on the woman's abdomen and limits how far the man's penis can extend into the vagina.

although the basic guide to intercourse during pregnancy is your own comfort, there are a few reasons your doctor may advise you to limit or avoid having intercourse:

- Past miscarriage or ***pretenm*** birth
- Infection
- Bleeding
- Pain
- Breaking of the amniotic sac or leaking amniotic fluid

Intercourse is not the only form of sexual expression. Other forms of expressing your sexuality can be equally satisfying. This is an area that you may wish to discuss with your doctor.

Whatever form of sexual expression you choose, it's best to stay with one steady partner. A monogamous relationship, in which both partners are faithful to each other, is more important now than ever. Women who have more than one sexual partner greatly increase their chances of getting a sexually transmitted disease. These diseases are dangerous for the mother and the fetus.

Harmful Agents

Teratogens are agents that can cause birth defects when a woman is exposed to them during pregnancy. Hazards can be posed by drugs that are prescribed, chemicals that occur in the environment or work place, or infections. These agents can interfere with the normal development of the fetus, resulting in physical and mental defects (other agents are suspect, but have not been proven to be harmful). Their effect depends on the fetus's stage of development when exposure occurred and the dosage received. Other substances, such as tobacco and illicit drugs, are harmful in different ways and should be avoided for the sake of your health and that of your baby.

Work-Related hazards

The risk of exposure to many of the substances that occur in the work place is not known. Scientific information is either lacking or conflicting. A few of the substances that can be found in the work place, however, are known to cause harm.

Heavy metals, such as lead and mercury, are teratogens. Lead is used in some industries. Tollbooth attendants and others who work on heavily traveled roads may also be exposed to high levels of lead.

Ionizing radiation is used to take X-rays of the internal organs to diagnose a problem. It can also be used in larger doses for treatment. In larger doses, such as those used to treat cancer, it can harm a fetus. Most women who work around radiation, however, are protected against exposure.

The radiation from color television sets, video display terminals (VDTs), and microwave ovens is known as nonionizing radiation. Persons working near these sources are not exposed to dangerous levels of radiation. In the last 10 Years, however, it has been suggested that the radiation from VDTs cause problems during pregnancy. VDTs, also called catholde-ray tubes (or CRTs), create both ionizing radiation, which is absorbed by the glass screen and nonionizing radiation, which can escape from the back of the unit. More studies are needed to determine for certain whether this affects the fetuses of pregnant VDT users.

If you think that you may be exposed to a hazardous agent through your work, talk to your employer about it. You may be able to be moved to another job on a temporary basis.

Medications

Any type of medicine can affect the fetus, and some can cause severe birth defects of other problems for the baby. Don't stop taking any medication prescribed by a doctor—the lack of treatment could be more harmful than the drug—but do seek medical advice.

Be sure that the doctor caring for you during pregnancy knows about any medical problems you may have. Tell him or her about any drugs other doctors have prescribed for you and whether you have any drug allergies. You may need to change the kind or amount of drug you take.

Not all drugs require a prescription. Products such as pain medicines (aspirin, acetaminophen, or ibuprofen), cold and allergy medicine, and some skin treatments are drugs, even though you can buy them in a drug store without a prescription. Over-the-counter drugs should not be taken during pregnancy without checking first with your doctor. Instructions that come with these over-the-counter drugs are usually not meant for a pregnant woman.

Agents that can Harm the Fetus

Agent	*Reasons Used*	*Effects*
Alcohol	Part of regular diet, social reasons, dependency	Growth and mental retardation
Androgens	To treat endometriosis	Genital abnormalities
Anticoagulants, eg, warfarin (Coumadin, Panwarfin) and dicumarol	To prevent blood clotting; used to prevent or treat thromboembolisms (clots blocking blood vessels)	Abnormalities in bones, cartilage, and eyes; central nervous system defects
Antithyroid drugs, eg, propylthiouracil, iodide, and methimazole (Tapazole)	To treat an overactive thyroid gland	Underactive or enlarged thyroid
Anticonvulsants, eg, phenytoin (Dilantin), trimethadione (Tridione), paramethadione (Paradione), valproic acid (Depakene)	To treat epilepsy and irregular heartbeat	Growth and meantal retardation, developmental abnormalities, neural tube defects
Chemotherapeutic drugs, eg, methotrexate (Mexate) and aminopterin	To treat cancer and psoriasis (skin disease)	Increased rate of miscarriage, various abnormalities
Diethylstilbestrol (DES)	To treat problems with menstruation, symptoms of menopause and breast cancer, and to stop milk production;	Abnormalities of cervix and uterus in females possible infertility in males and females
Lead	Industies involving lead smelting paint manufacture and use, printing, ceramics, glass manufacturing, and pottery glazing	Increased rate of miscarriage and stillbirths
Lithium	To treat the manic part of manic-depressive disorders	Congenital heart disease
Organic mercury	Exposure through eating contaminated food	Brain disorders
Isotretinoin (Accutane)	Treatment for cystic acne	Increased rate of miscarriage, developmental abnormalities
Streptomycin	An antibiotic used to treat tuberculosis	Hearing loss
Tetracycline	An antibiotic used to treat a wide variety of infections	Underdevelopment of tooth enamel, incorporation of tetracycline into bone

Agent	Reasons Used	Effects
Thalidomide	Previously used as a sedative and a sleep aid	Growth deficiencies, other abnormalities
X-ray therapy	Medical treatment of disorders such as cancer	Growth and mental retardation

Illicit Drugs

The life style that often goes with the use of illicit drugs often makes it difficult to pinpoint their effects during pregnancy. It is known, however, that drug users are more likely to have problems during pregnancy that place their babies at risk. The effects of drugs can be so harmful that even occasional users are at risk.

Marijuana is the illicit drug that is used most often. Women who are moderate or heavy users (two to five uses per week) tend to deliver early, and their babies are often small. Marijuana can be retained in the body for long periods, leading to prolonged fetal exposure, and it contains carbon monoxide, a gas that could keep the fetus from receiving enough oxygen.

Cocaine, the second most often used illicit drug, is especially dangerous during pregnancy. It can be snorted, injected, or smoked in a highly purified and addictive form known as crack. Cocaine abuse is more harmful than any other substance abuse in pregnancy. Pregnant women who use cocaine have a 25% higher chance of having a preterm birth. Their babies are at risk for being small for their age and are often more irritable and fussy. Cocaine can cause the mother to have a heart attack and could cause death of the fetus. Recent studies suggest that even babies who survive being exposed to cocaine during pregnancy will have long-lasting physical, behavioral, and emotional problems.

Other illicit drugs, such as heroin, methadone, and phencyclidine (PCP or angel dust), can be addictive to the baby as well as the mother. When these babies are born, they must go through withdrawal from the drug.

Addictions can be hard to quit. Pregnancy may give you extra incentive to try. If you want to stop using illegal drugs, talk to your doctor. He or she can give you more information about the effects of these drugs on your fetus and can refer you to a treatment program.

You should try to stop taking any drugs as soon as possible. The fetus's organs form during the first ***trimester***, and using drugs during this time can cause serious damage to these organs. Cutting down on or stopping drug use anytime in pregnancy, however, does provide some benefits.

Smoking

When a pregnant woman smokes, she risks not only her own health but that of her baby. smoking hurts the baby before, during, and after birth. Each puff exposes the fetus to harmful chemicals. Carbon monoxide travels to the fetus's blood. This lowers the amount of oxygen to both the mother and the fetus. Nicotine crosses the ***placenta*** (which connects mother and fetus) and can cause the fetal blood vessels to constrict so that less oxygen and nourishment reach the fetus.

Smoking increases a woman's risk of complications during pregnancy.

Pregnant smokers are more apt to have have vaginal bleeding during pregnancy. They are also more likely to have a miscarriage, ***stillbirth,*** or preterm baby (born before 37 weeks). On the average, a smoker's baby weighs 1/2 pound less than a nonsmoker's baby and is about 1/2 inch shorter in body length. Low birth weight raises the baby's chances of being born early and needing special care. ***Sudden infant death syndrome (SIDS)*** occurs more than twice as often among babies of smoking mothers.

The sooner you quit, the better it will be for your baby. If you stop smoking during the early months of your pregnancy, your chance of having a low-birth-weight baby will be close to that of a non-smoker. Almost one-fourth of all pregnant women quit smoking while they are pregnant. If you cannot stop smoking, you can still help your fetus by smoking as little as possible. If you can quit during pregnancy, you can quit for a lifetime, and it will be a healthier one.

Alcohol

About 60% of American women drink alcoholic beverages. There is a difference between alcohol *use* and alcohol *abuse.* Some people have one or tow drinks on various occasions—this is alcohol use. Others may drink daily or in binges (drinking a large amount of alcohol in a short time)—this is alcohol abuse. The amount of alcohol that separates use from abuse is not clearly defined.

When a pregnant woman drinks alcohol, it quickly reaches the fetus through the bloodstream. The same level of alcohol that goes through the mother's bloodstream also goes through the fetus's. A number of studies have been done on infants born to women who drank heavily during pregnancy. Many of the infants were born with a strong pattern of physical, mental, and behavioral problems. This group of problems is called fetal alcohol syndrome.

Babies that had the syndrome were shorter and lighter in weight than normal babies and did`not catch up, even after special care was provided. They also had small heads; abnormal features of the face, head, joints, and limbs; heart defects; and poor control of movements. most were mentally retarded and showed a number of behavioral problems, including hyperactivity, extreme nervousness, and poor attention span. Some of the infants were born with all of these problems; others showed signs of only some of them.

Other factors—cigarette smoking, use of other drugs, poor diet, problems handling stress—may well play a role in fetal alcohol syndrome. But alcohol itself appears to be the one common agent in all cases. Other factors alone cannot account for the damage.

It appears that the more a mother drinks during pregnancy, the greater the danger to the fetus. The fetus is especially at risk early in pregnancy, when all of the major body systems are being developed. Alcohol increases the risk of having a miscarriage at this time. The risk is about twice as high in pregnancies complicated by maternal drinking, although perhaps only among women who drink heavily.

One of the questions asked most often about alcohol and pregnancy is whether there is a safe level of alcohol intake. Does the woman who drinks only once in a while put her baby in danger? There is no evidence that an occasional drink is harmful. Women who have an occasional drink seem to have babies with no more problems than those women who drink rarely or not at all.

Moderation is the key. Avoid binges and daily drinking. That type of drinking is more dangerous. Even if you don't binge and you believe your drinking is moderate, it's still best to try to cut down. Reducing intake anytime during pregnancy can be beneficial.

It is hard to state how much alcohol puts the fetus at risk. Each fetus may be affected differently. It is best to cut down gradually over a 6-month period before you become pregnant. Because it isn't known how much alcohol is harmful, the safest course is to drink alcohol rarely or not at all during pregnancy. It's just one more way to change your life style in order to increase your chances of having a healthy, normal baby.

Do You Have a Drinking Problem?

Sometimes it can be hard to tell the difference between alcohol use and alcohol abuse. Experts in treating alcohol abuse use the CAGE questions to help them find out whether a person has a drinking problem:

C Have you ever felt you ought to **cut down** on your drinking?

A Have people **annoyed** you by criticizing your drinking?

G Have you ever felt bad or **guilty** about your drinking?

E Have you ever had a drink first thing in the morning to steady your nerves or to get rid of a hangover? Ever had an **eye-opener?**

If you answer "yes" to any of these questions, or if you notice an increased tolerance to drinking, you may have a problem with alcohol. Talk to your doctor about your drinking habits. He or she can give you more information and refer you for counseling or treatment.

The Battered Woman

Abuse of women by their male partners—physical, sexual, or emotional abuse—is one of America's most widespread health problems. It can occur regardless of socioeconomic or ethnic group, race, age, or religion. The consequences of this abuse are serious. About 20% of the visits made by women to emergency rooms are for injuries related to abuse. Over one-third of female murder victims are killed by their male partners. Children may also be affected, because men who abuse their partners often also abuse their children.

Abuse often begins or increases during pregnancy, putting both the mother and the fetus at risk. During pregnancy, the abuser is more likely to direct his blows at the woman's breasts and abdomen. Dangers to the fetus include miscarriage, low birth weight, and direct injury from blows to the mother's abdomen. Sometimes, though, abuse decreases during pregnancy. In fact, some women feel safe only when they are carrying a child. This can lead to repeated pregnancies as a way of escaping abuse.

There are better ways of dealing with abuse, though. First, realize that you are not to blame for your partner's actions. Abusers blame their victims, but it is not your fault. He and he alone is the cause of his actions. Second, tell someone you trust about your situation—a close friend, doctor or nurse, counselor, or a clergy member. Letting someone else know can be a relief, and the person you tell can help you get in touch with support services such as crisis hot lines, domestic violence programs, legal aid services, or shelters for battered women and children. Counseling can help you to understand the situation and to make a decision about what to do.

The next step is ensuring your safety and the safety of any children you have. Make a rapid-action plan that will allow you and your children to level quickly, if needed. Some steps you may want to follow include:

- Pack a suitcase to store with a friend or neighbor. Include a change of clothes for you and your children and an extra set of keys to the house and car.
- Keep important items in a safe place so you can take them with you on short notice—prescription medicines; identification such as birth certificates, social

security cards, and driver's license; cash, a checkbook, savings account book, and credit cards; and a special toy for each child.

- Know exactly where you will go and how to get there at any time of the day.
- Know what you will do if you can't escape the violence—to to the doctor or emergency room, tell the doctor how you were hurt, and ask for a copy of your medical record in case you want to file charges later.
- Call the police—physical abuse is a crime, even if you are living with or married to the abuser.

Learn to recognize the signs of impending danger so you can use your exit plan to avoid a violent incident. These can include your male partner having a weapon or threatening to use one, threatening or hurting children or other members of the family, forcing you to have sex, or showing less guilt and remorse after he is violent.

No one deserves to be abused: not you, not your fetus, and not your children. If your male partner has begun or continues to abuse you, talk to someone and start taking steps to end the violence.

Work

Today more than 51 million women make up almost half of America's work force. Of these, more than 1 million become pregnant each year. Many of these women work until a short time before delivery and return to work within weeks or months of the baby's birth. This trend, along with a growing awareness of on-the-job health and safety, has prompted women, doctors, and employers to ask a number of questions that have no easy answers: Is it safe for a pregnant woman to work? How long, under what conditions, and with what effects can she continue to work?

If your job is strenuous or requires a lot of standing or walking, your doctor may ask you to cut back on work hours, transfer to less strenuous work, or stop working a few weeks before delivery. Your doctor may also advise you to stop working if you have certain diseases, have given birth to more than one premature baby, have a history of miscarriages, or are expecting more than one baby. Otherwise, if you are a normal, healthy woman—with an uncomplicated pregnancy and a normally developing fetus—and you work in a job that presents no greater hazards than those in daily life, you can usually work until your due date.

Pregnancy-Related Disability

Having a disability means that you are not able to work because of physical problems that could interfere with your ability to perform your usual duties. Only you and your doctor can decide whether your pregnancy is partially or totally disabling. A disability may fall into any of three categories:

1. *Disability of the pregnancy itself.* Some women suffer side effects such as nausea, vomiting, indigestion problems, dizziness, and swollen legs and ankles during pregnancy. Your doctor should reevaluate these minor problems at regular intervals.

2. *Disability related to complications.* More serious complications, such as infection, bleeding, or early rupture of the amniotic sac, may cause disability. Also, medical conditions you had before becoming pregnant, such as heart disease, diabetes, or high blood pressure, may be disabling during pregnancy.

3. *Disability related to job exposure.* Some disabilities may be job related, linked with such factors as exposure to high levels of toxic substances.

If your doctor decides that your pregnancy is disabling, you may request a letter to verify to your employer that you are eligible for disability benefits. Likewise, if your doctor says you are able to keep working, your employer may request you (or you may choose) to submit a letter from your doctor stating so.

Disability Benefits for Pregnant Employees

Employee maternity policies vary widely from company to company and state to state. Only about 40% of employed women in the United States are entitled to paid 6-week disability leave for childbirth. Others must use sick leave and vacation time or take time off without pay.

The Pregnancy Discrimination Act, passed by Congress in 1978, requires employers offering medical disability compensation to treat pregnancy-related disabilities in the same manner as all other disabilities. It means that if you are temporarily unable to work because of pregnancy, your employer must give you the same rights as other employees temporarily disabled by illness or accident. If you are partially disabled by pregnancy and your employer regularly assigns lighter work to other partially disabled workers, the same must be done for you. Unfortunately, many employers offer no disability benefits at all and therefore are not obligated to provide maternity leave.

If no disability plan is offered where you work, you may qualify for unemployment or temporary disability benefits from your state. To find out whether your state offers benefits and how to qualify, contact your local unemployment office.

Pregnant women can usually keep doing the physical activities they are used to doing. Heavy lifting, climbing, carrying, and other efforts requiring agility and stamina may cause discomfort for some. These and long hours may pose a risk.

The first few months of pregnancy may bring periods of dizziness, nausea, fatigue, and heat sensitivity that can increase the risk of accidents. Toward the end of pregnancy, you become more vulnerable to falls because your body balance changes with your increase in weight and abdomen size. Also, because women tire more easily when pregnant, even those in the best physical condition will find strenuous labor more tiring than usual.

At home, housework and child care duties don't stop during pregnancy and can also be strenuous work. More responsibilities may need to be shared at this time with your partner or others to ensure you are getting enough rest.

Your Rights as an Employee

The 1978 Pregnancy Act is an amendment to the Civil Rights Act of 1964. This act requires your employer to offer the same medical disability compensation for pregnancy-related disabilities as is offered for other disabilities.

The Occupational Safety and Health Administration (OSHA) in Washington, DC (phone: 202–634–7460), administered under the Department of labor, was created under the Occupational Safety and Health Act of 1970. OSHA sets and enforces standards requiring employers to provide a work place free from recognized hazards causing, or likely to cause, death or serious physical harm and to provide information to employees about dangerous chemicals and substances. State and municipal statutes also give employees and unions the right to request the names of chemicals and other substances used in the work place. At the request of an employee, union, or health care provided, OSHA representatives will perform work place inspections.

The National Institute for Occupational Safety and Health (NIOSH) in Atlanta (phone: 404–331–2396) operates under the Department of Health and Human Services. While OSHA is in charge of regulation in the work place, NIOSH is responsible for research—identifying hazards, figuring out ways to control them, and recommending federal standards to limit the dangers. At the request of an employee, union, or health care provider, NIOSH investigates health and safety standards in the work place.

Travel

Travel during pregnancy is generally safe if you make certain allowances and preparations. The most comfortable time in pregnancy for most women to travel is during the second trimester (14–28 weeks of gestation). By this time, your body has adjusted to pregnancy, and you probably have more energy. Morning sickness is usually no longer a problem during these months, and the rate of complications is at its lowest.

The best method of transportation when you are pregnant is very often the one you enjoy most. There are some hints that apply no matter what type of transportation you choose:

- You will be more comfortable if you stop frequently and walk around. Try to walk around and stretch every hour and a half.
- Be sure to wear comfortable clothing that doesn't bind.
- Take some crackers or other light snacks with you to help prevent nausea.
- Traveling can upset your stomach and disrupt your sleeping habits and your health. Do not take any medications—either prescription drugs or over-the-counter preparations—without checking with your doctor. This includes anti-motion-sickness pills and laxatives.
- Take a copy of your prenatal record with you.
- Ask your doctor to recommend another doctor who can care for you at your new location if you plan to be away from home for an extended time.
- Check with your doctor about the chance of premature labor if you plan to travel very late in pregnancy.

Although travel during pregnancy is considered safe in most cases, it is not recommended for women who have serious health problems that need special medical care. If you are unsure about whether travel is safe for you, ask your doctor.

The Right Way to Wear a Safety Belt

For the best protection, you should wear a lap-shoulder belt throughout your pregnancy every time you travel in a car, including during your ride to the hospital for the birth of your baby. Some cars have only lap belts in the back seat. If a lap belt is all that is available, use it.

Place the lower part of the lap-shoulder belt under your abdomen, as low as possible, and against your upper thighs. Never place the belt above your abdomen, because this could cause major injures in a crash. Position the upper part of the belt between your breasts. Adjust both the upper and lower parts of the lap- shoulder belt as snugly as possible.

The belt should cross your shoulder without chafing your neck. Never slip the upper part of the belt off your shoulder. Safety belts worn too loosely or too high on the abdomen can cause broken ribs or injuries to your abdomen. But more damage is caused when they aren't used at all.

Foreign Travel: Let the Traveler Beware

If you are thinking about taking a trip out of the country, discuss your plans with your doctor. He or she can help you decide whether foreign travel would be safe for you, and if so, what steps you should take in advance.

Traveling to other countries exposes you to diseases that are not common in the United States. Natives of a country are used to the organisms found in the food and water, but the same organisms can make a visitor ill. This is true whether you travel to cities or rural areas.

Although traveler's diarrhea may be a minor nuisance to a nonpregnant traveler, it is a greater concern for a pregnant women. The best way to avoid getting diarrhea is by avoiding contaminated food and water. Iodine used to purify water may not be safe for pregnant women. Drink only pure bottled water, bottled soft drinks, hot tea, or broth. Don't use ice in your drinks, and avoid using glasses that could have been washed in contaminated water. Instead, drink out of the bottle or use paper cups. Avoid fresh fruits and vegetables unless they have been cooked or can be peeled.

If you do get diarrhea, drink plenty of pure water and other fluids. Do not take any medicine without checking with a doctor first. There are some medicines safe for treating diarrhea during pregnancy that a doctor can prescribe.

Malaria is a tropical infection passed on by mosquito bites. It produces flu-like symptoms and anemia. Complications of malaria are more common in pregnant women, and malaria increases the risk of miscarriage, stillbirth, and small babies. Avoiding mosquito bites by wearing long-sleeved clothing and using mosquito netting, bug repellent, or lotion is the best way to avoid malaria. Although no drug completely protects you against malaria, chloroquine is effective in preventing and treating most cases. It is safe for use in pregnancy. You must start taking it before you travel and continue afterwards for a few weeks. You should not plan to travel to areas where there are mosquitoes that carry strains of malaria that are resistant to chloroquine (such as East Africa and Thailand), because there is no other safe drug that prevents malaria.

Immunization is often not required by law for travel, but depending on where you plan to go, it may be a good idea.

Ideally, vaccines should be given before you become pregnant, but some can be given during pregnancy. As a rule, though, live vaccines should not be given during pregnancy. You and your doctor will need to decide whether the risks of a disease are greater than the risks of its vaccine. In some cases it may be best to postpone a trip until fter pregnancy.

By Land

Traveling by car can be a good choice, especially if you're traveling a short-to-medium distance. If you travel by car, be sure to wear your seat belt. Some women worry that the belt will squeeze the fetus if the car stops quickly or if there is an impact, but this is very unlikely. Inside the uterus, which is protected by muscles, organs, and bones, the fetus is cushioned in a fluid-filled sac. Studies have shown that in nearly 100% of car crashes, the fetus recovers quickly from any pressure the seat belt exerts and suffers no lasting injury. The risk of *not* wearing a seat belt include being thrown from the car or receiving a concussion, an injury to the brain that is caused by a hard blow.

These risks are much more serious than any from wearing a seat belt.

Buses may not allow much room to move around, and stops will be farther apart than if you were driving. When traveling long distances, trains may allow you more freedom of movement than buses.

By Air

Flying is generally safe during pregnancy. Airlines in the United States usually allow pregnant women to fly up to 36 weeks of pregnancy. Commercial airplanes are pressurized, but many private planes are not. It is best to avoid altitudes greater than 7,000–9,000 feet in unpressurized airplanes.

When flying, try to get an aisle seat (in the forward part of the cabin for a more stable ride) so you can get up and move around and have easy access to the bathroom. You should try to stand and walk in the aisle or do leg lifts. Eat lightly to avoid airsickness. Special meals are available on many flights if you order in advance. The metal detectors used for airport security checks are not harmful to the fetus.

By Sea

Boat cruises can be a slow, often relaxing way to travel. Still, travel by boat may present special concerns. If you are thinking about taking a cruise, you might want to discuss some of these issues with your doctor:

- Medicine you can take for seasickness
- Distance from medical care while the cruise is on the open sea
- Special diet concerns

Questions to Consider....

- Can I continue my present exercise program?
- Do my partner and I need to change our sexual practices during pregnancy?
- What can I do to remove myself and my fetus from harmful agents or situations?
- Is it safe for me to work while I'm pregnant? How long should I plan to be off work?
- Should I alter my travel plan while I'm pregnant?

39

Changes During Pregnancy

As your fetus grows, your uterus increases to about 1,000 times its original size. This amount of growth, centered in one area, affects other parts of your body. Many of the changes in your body that occur during pregnancy are triggered by hormones (substances produced by the body to control the functions of various organs) that nurture the fetus and prepare for childbirth. These changes have a physical and emotional impact and may cause discomforts. Some may occur only in the early weeks of pregnancy. Others may occur only as you get closer to the end of your pregnancy. Still others may appear early, then go away, only to return again later. This is normal and usually does not mean that anything is wrong. Every woman's pregnancy is unique, as are her responses to it. Share your concerns, discomforts, and questions with your doctor, who may be able to suggest things you can do to make yourself feel more comfortable.

Physical Changes

Backache

Backache is one of the most common complaints during pregnancy. It is usually caused by the strain put on the back muscles by your growing uterus and by changes in your posture. Here are some suggestions to help lessen back pain:

- Wear low-heeled (but not flat) shoes.
- Avoid lifting heavy objects or children.
- Do not bend over from the waist to pick things up—squat down, bending your knees and keeping your back straight.
- Place one foot on a stool or box when you have to stand for long periods.
- Arrange things at home and at work at a comfortable level, so that you don't have to bend or stretch too much.
- Check that your bed is firm enough. If it is too soft, placing a board between the mattress and box spring (have someone help you) can be helpful.
- Sleep on your side with one knee bent and your upper leg supported on a pillow.
- Apply heat, cold, or pressure to the painful area.
- Do special exercises—ask your doctor or nurse for specific instructions.

Breast Changes

Starting early in pregnancy, your breasts undergo many changes to prepare for breast-feeding your baby. In fact, changes to your breasts may be one of the first signs that your are pregnant. By 6–8 weeks of pregnancy, your breasts will be noticeably larger. This is because the fat layer of your breasts is thickening, and the number of milk glands is increasing.

Your breasts will continue to grow in size and weight throughout the first **trimes-*ter.*** Changes in breast size may be more obvious in women with small breasts and less obvious in women with large breasts. Your breasts will feel firm and tender. As your breasts grow, wearing a good bra that fits well will provide you with support. To fuel the growth of your breasts, their blood supply increases, and the veins close to the surface become larger and more noticeable. You may feel some tingling, or your breasts may be sensitive to touch.

Also early in pregnancy, your nipples and ***areolas*** (the darker skin around your nipples) will darken. Your nipples may project out more now. This helps your baby firmly latch on to your breast if you breast-feed. Your areolas also grow larger. On the surface of the areolas also grow larger. On the surface of the areolas are small glands called Montgomery tubercles. They produce an oily substance that helps protect the nipple from cracking or drying out. The Montgomery tubercles now become raised and bumpy.

If you plan to breast-feed, you may want to prepare your nipples. To toughen the area where your baby will suck, you can expose your breasts to air, wear a nursing bra with the flaps down, or gently rub your nipples with a washcloth. Soaps or creams should not be used.

Some women's nipples do not project out but sink inward (***retracted nipple***). If you have retracted nipples and you plan to breast-feed, your doctor may recommend that you try massaging the nipples so they protrude more. You can also gently pull on either side of the areola with your forefingers. In time, this will also cause the nipple to stick out.

By about 12–14 weeks of pregnancy, your breasts may begin producing ***colostrum,*** the fluid that will feed your baby for his or her first few days before your milk comes in. This doesn't happen in every woman, so don't be concerned if you don't produce colostrum before delivery. Colostrum contains water, proteins, minerals, and ***antibodies*** that protect your baby from disease.

Early in pregnancy, the colostrum will probably be thick and yellow, but toward the end of pregnancy, it will become pale and nearly colorless. Colostrum may leak from your breasts by itself or if you massage your breasts. It also tends to leak out during times of sexual excitement.

Breathing Problems

As the fetus grows inside your uterus, the uterus expands and takes up more room in your abdomen. In the third trimester, by about 31–34 weeks of pregnancy, the uterus has grown so large that it presses the digestive organs and the diaphragm (a flat, strong muscle that aids in breathing) up toward the lungs. Because the lungs do not have as much room to expand as before, you may find you are short of breath. Even if you feel you are not getting enough air, you need not worry about the fetus. it will get all the oxygen it needs.

A few weeks before you give birth, the fetus's head will move down in the uterus, or "drop" and press against the cervix. This usually happens between 36–38 weeks of pregnancy in women who have not been pregnant before, but in women who have already been pregnant, it may not happen until the beginning of labor. When the fetus drops, you will find it easier to breathe, because the uterus will not be pressing as much on your other organs.

If being short of breath makes you uncomfortable, here are some ideas to try:

- Take life a little more slowly, so your heart and lungs don't have to work so hard.
- Sit up straight.

- Sleep propped up.
- Ask your doctor or a childbirth educator about breathing exercises to help you breathe more deeply.

Constipation

At least half of all pregnant women seem to have problems with constipation. One reason for this may be changes in hormones that slow the movement of food through the digestive tract. During the last part of pregnancy, pressure on your rectum from your uterus may add to the problem. Here are some suggestion that may help:

- Drink plenty of liquids—at least eight glasses each day, including fruit juices such as prune juice.
- Eat food high in fiber, such as raw fruits and vegetables and bran cereals.
- Exercise daily–just walking is fine.

Cramps

In the last 3 months of pregnancy, you may find that you have leg cramps. Although it was once though the cramps were caused by a problem with the amount of calcium in your diet, this is no longer thought to be true. Stretching your legs before going to bed can help relieve cramps, but avoid pointing your toes when stretching or exercising.

Fatigue

You may feel tired often during pregnancy—especially during the first and last 3 months. The remedy for fatigue relies on common sense: get enough exercise and rest (including naps) and eat a well-balanced diet.

Frequent Urination

There is usually a desire to urinate frequently during the first 3 months of pregnancy. It is mainly caused by the pressure of the growing uterus on the bladder, the organ in which urine is stored. Even though your bladder may be nearly empty, this pressure produces the same kind of sensation as when the bladder is full of urine.

Kegel Exercises

Kegel exercises, or perineal exercises, are used to strengthen the muscles that surround the openings of the urethra, vagina, and anus. Your doctor or nurse can help you learn to perform these exercises. If you contract these muscles for about 3 seconds, 12–15 times in a row, at least six times a day, in time you will begin to notice some improvement in your ability to hold your urine.

As your uterus grows and rises higher into your abdomen, the symptoms may disappear. In the last month or so, though, urinary frequency may return as the fetus drops into the pelvis and again presses against the bladder. Especially toward the end of pregnancy, you may find that the need to urinate wakes you up several times during the night. If the pressure of the uterus on the bladder causes you to leak some urine, there are special exercises called Kegel exercises that can help strengthen the muscles around the urethra (the tube that carries urine from the bladder out of the body). If you have pain when you urinate or if you often feel you need to urinate right away, you should talk to your doctor. You could have an infection.

Groin or Lower Abdominal Pain

As the uterus grows, the round ligaments (bands of fibrous tissue along both sides of the uterus) that support it are pulled and stretched. You may occasionally feel this as either sharp pains in your abdomen, usually on the side, or a dull ache. The pains are most common between 18–24 weeks. to help prevent these pains, avoid quick changes of position, especially when you are turning at the waist. When you do feel a pain, bend toward it to relieve it. Resting and changing your position also seem to help.

Hemorrhoids

Very often pregnant women who are constipated also have hemorrhoids. Hemorrhoids are varicose (or swollen) veins of the rectum. They are often painful. Straining during bowel movements and having very hard stools may increase the severity of hemorrhoids and sometimes may cause them to protrude from the rectum.

Do not take drugstore cures while you are pregnant without first checking with your doctor. Several things can help give relief or avoid the problem in the first place:

- Avoid constipation.
- Eat a high-fiber diet.
- Drink plenty of liquids.
- Exercise.

Indigestion

Indigestion is commonly called heartburn, but it does not mean that anything is wrong with your heart. It is a burning sensation that is first felt in the stomach and seems to rise up into the throat. It occurs when digested food from your stomach, which contains acid, is pushed up into your esophagus (the tube leading from the throat to the stomach). Because liquids are food and take up space in your stomach, they can also contribute to the problem.

Changes that take place in your body during pregnancy may worsen indigestion. Changes in your hormone levels slow digestion and relax the muscle that keeps the digested food and acids in you stomach, preventing it from entering the esophagus. In addition, your growing uterus presses up on your stomach.

To help relieve heartburn, try the following:

- Eat five or six small meals a day instead of two or three large ones.
- Avoid foods that cause gas, such as spicy or greasy foods.
- Sit up while eating.
- Wait an hour after eating before lying down and do not eat before bedtime.
- Wait 2 hours after eating before exercising.

Do not take any medications unless you first check with your docto64XThis includes antacids and baking soda.

Insomnia

This problem is especially evident in the last months of pregnancy, when your abdomen has grown so large that a comfortable position can be hard to find. Several remedies can help you to get the rest you need:

- A warm bath at bedtime
- Relaxation techniques learned in childbirth classes
- Lying on your side with a pillow supporting your abdomen and another between your legs
- Short periods of rest during the day

Nausea and Vomiting

Most often caused by changes in hormones, nausea and vomiting are common complaints during the first 3 months of pregnancy. Nausea and vomiting sometimes return late is pregnancy. They are usually called morning sickness, but they can occur any time during the day, especially when the stomach is empty. There are some things you can do to feel more comfortable:

- Arise slowly when you wake up and sit on the side of the bed for a few minutes.
- Eat dry toast, crackers, a peeled apple, or a plain potato (peeled and cooked).
- Eat five or six small meals each day–try to avoid having your stomach completely empty.
- Avoid unpleasant odors when possible.
- Avoid drinking citrus juice, water, milk, coffee, and tea.

If nausea or vomiting becomes severe, notify your doctor. always check with your doctor before taking any medication.

Numbness and Tingling

As the uterus increases in size and rests on certain nerves, numbness and tingling in the legs, toes, and sometimes in the arms may occur. This is usually not serious and will go away after the baby is born.

Skin Changes

The different amounts of hormones in your body often contribute to some normal changes on certain areas of your skin. Some women notice brownish, uneven blotches around the eyes and over the nose and cheekbones. This is called ***chloasma***. These marks usually disappear or fade after delivery, when hormone levels go back to normal. Being in the sunlight tends to increase these skin changes.

Many women notice the darkening of a line running from the top to the bottom of the abdomen. This is called the ***linea nigra***. Others may notice streaks or stretch marks on the abdomen and breasts as they grow during pregnancy. This is caused by the skin tissue stretching to support the extra weight. There is no way to prevent stretch marks, but they will slowly fade after pregnancy.

Swelling

A certain amount of swelling (celled ***edema***) seems to be normal during pregnancy. It occurs most often in the legs, and usually disappears in the morning. Swelling can begin during the last few months of pregnancy. It occurs most often in the legs, and usually disappears in the morning. Swelling can begin during the last few months of pregnancy, and it may occur more often in the summer. Let your doctor know if you have swelling in your hands or face, because this may mean that there is another problem. Never take medicines for swelling unless your doctor has prescribed them. You can help the swelling in your legs go down by trying these suggestions:

- Elevate your legs when possible.
- Rest in bed on your side, preferably your left side.
- Do not wear anything that binds your legs, such as tight garters or bands around stockings or socks.
- Exercise regularly, especially walking, swimming, or riding an exercise bike.
- Wear support pantyhose or stockings.

Varicose Veins

Varicose, or swollen, veins appear most often in the legs but can also appear near the vulva and vagina. They are causes by pressure from the weight of your uterus on your veins and frequently develop if you must stand or sit for long periods of time. This condition is usually not serious but can be uncomfortable and may cause aching, sore legs.

Some of these suggestions may help:

- Elevate your legs when possible.
- Lie on the floor with your legs raised on a small footstool or several pillows. Tuck a pillow under one hip so that you are not absolutely flat on the floor.
- If your job requires much sitting, stand up and move around frequently to help your circulation.
- Try not to stand for long periods of time.
- Do not wear anything that binds your legs, such as tight garters or bands around stockings or socks.
- Wear support stockings, or your doctor can recommend special elastic stockings.

Emotional Changes

Pregnancy is a time of not only physical changes but also emotional changes. Although many women feel very good during pregnancy, the increa[illegible] hormones that enable a woman's body to maintain and support the pregnancy may also result in mood swings, especially during the first 3 months. Extreme tiredness in early and late pregnancy may also make you feel irritable or depressed. Regular periods of rest and relaxation will help you emotional as well as physical well-being.

Mood Swings

Perhaps the worst thing about mood swings is that they are unpredictable. A minor problem may not bother you one day and may have you in tears the next. Not knowing how you will react to a situation makes it hard on you, your family, and your friends. These unpredictable changes are often caused by the changes in your levels of hormones. These changes are not something you can control, so don't blame yourself if you are often teary or short- tempered.

The hormones that are needed to support your pregnancy form a complex system: levels of some hormones are rising, while levels of others are falling. These changes are needed to bring about all the different stages of your pregnancy. When hormones control so many functions in the body, it makes sense that constantly changing levels would affect you.

Although pregnancy is mostly a happy time, you may feel sad or worried now and then. These feelings are normal and are caused partly by the changes in your hormone levels. Fatigue can also cause or worsen feelings of sadness. Especially during the last few weeks of pregnancy, you may feel tired often. The newness of being pregnant has worn off, and the extra weight you are carrying may make you feel heavy and slow. These feelings will usually pass quickly after delivery.

Anxiety

Pregnant women and their partners often have many fears and worries about the pregnancy, labor and delivery, the effect of a child on their lives, and whether they will be good parents. Usually there is nothing to worry about, but these feelings may prompt you to make decisions and take actions that will help things go more smoothly.

Many parents-to-be worry that their child will not be normal. By far, most children are born healthy. You know that you can take steps to help ensure a healthy child. These include eating right; resting and exercising; avoiding drugs, alcohol, and a high-risk sexual life style; and receiving early and regular prenatal care. You can also take advantage of any tests your doctor recommends that can show the health of the fetus.

Women also are often anxious about labor and delivery, especially if they have not given birth before. Learning what to expect can be a big help. You may fear the pain and think that you won't be able to stand it. You can prepare for labor and the birth of your child by learning about methods that can help relieve pain. These methods for breathing and relaxing are taught in childbirth preparation classes. Different kinds of pain medication also can help you during labor and birth. Even if you hadn't planned on using pain medication, don't feel as though you have failed if you need it. You cannot be a good participant in the birth of your baby if you are in a great deal of pain. Medication can help ease the pain enough so that you can do your part as you practiced.

Although all the instruction you've received about giving birth may have convinced you otherwise, having a baby is a natural event. There are no grades given for having a baby. If you plan to use childbirth preparation techniques, you may fear that you will forget them. Practice will make them second nature.

If your labor is very long or if the size or position of your fetus presents a problem, you may need some help in childbirth. If instruments such as ***forceps*** are used, or if your doctor decides you need to deliver by a cesarean birth instead of vaginally, do not think that you have field. Sometimes things don't go according to plan. You and your partner will want to be flexible and do what is best for you and the baby, even if it hasn't been rehearsed ahead of time.

Every parent is new to parenthood at some time and must learn how to care for, feed, and bathe a baby. If this is your first child, usually a nurse or someone at the hospital will be able to help you learn the basics about caring for the baby before you go home. Once you're home, your family and friends will probably also give you their own advice.

There are as many different ways of raising a baby as there are children. You will find the one that is right for you. Talking to other mothers can help relieve you of some fears and give you practical tips you can use. There are also a number of good books and classes on child care. Your pediatrician, the baby's doctor, may be able to recommend some for you.

Having a baby will mean big changes in your life. It doesn't mean, however, that you will be trapped or that the baby will take over your lives. You and your partner can still enjoy activities you shared before you became pregnant, and can now alter them to include your baby.

Body Image

When you are pregnant, your body undergoes nearly a total remaking—all the more amazing because of how fast it happens. It can be hard for your mind to keep up with your body's changes. As your breasts enlarge, your waistline begins disappearing, and your abdomen grows larger, you may have very mixed feelings. On the one hand, this change is an exciting, very visible reminder of the new life growing inside you. There will probably be days, though, when you'll just feel fat and wonder if you'll ever have your old body back. It is normal to have mixed feelings about the changes in your body. Exercise may help you feel better about how you look and, after delivery, can help you get back in shape.

Your Partner

Both you and your partner will have many adjustments to make throughout your pregnancy. Your old roles are changing, and you need to work to adapt to your new roles. You both may spend much of your time thinking about the baby, and you need to remember to make time for each other. Try to be understanding of each other. Pregnancy is a special time for a couple, but it can also cause stress and strains in your relationship because so much is changing. Being in a supportive relationship eases the course of pregnancy and the move into parenthood.

Because all the physical changes of pregnancy are happening to you, it is easy to forget that your partner is a part of the pregnancy, too. He is making his own adjustments, getting ready to be a father. Make a special effort to include him in things. Don't shut him out. Let him be a part of your pregnancy plans. He should attend childbirth classes with you and join you in exercising, buying clothes for the baby, and getting the baby's space ready.

Your sexual feelings about each other may also change. It is a good idea to talk to each other, so that you understand how your partner is feeling and so that he understands your concerns. Talking can bring you closer and help avoid hurt feelings and loneliness due to misunder-standings. Some couples find that pregnancy brings them together and that they feel closer than ever.

Because of your increased hormone levels and the fact that your body may be more sensitive to touch, you may be more easily aroused. Many men and women find a pregnant woman's larger breasts and rounded abdomen very sensuous. Other couples find that it is harder to enjoy sex now. Especially during the first and third trimesters, when you are more likely to feel nauseated and tired, sex may seem like a big bother. Your thoughts may focus on the baby, and your sexual feelings may be pushed aside. You or your partner may worry about injuring the baby if you have sex. In most cases, this will not happen, but for more guidelines, see "Sex," Chapter 7, and ask your doctor.

Questions to Consider...

- What can I do to relieve the discomforts of pregnancy?
- What if morning sickness doesn't go away or becomes very severe?
- Do I need to do anything to prepare my breasts for breast-feeding?

- Is it all right to take any over-the-counter medications if I feel really uncomfortable?
- If I develop varicose veins or hemorrhoids, will they go away after the baby is born?
- Are there ways in which my partner can become more involved in the pregnancy?

40

Special-Care Pregnancies

Pregnancy puts new demands on a woman's body. It can alter the course of some medical conditions a woman may have before pregnancy, and some conditions can affect the course of pregnancy. A woman with such a medical condition can have a healthy baby. An extra effort will be required, however, so that the woman's general health and her pregnancy can be followed more closely.

If you have a condition that could complicate your pregnancy, your doctor may order additional tests and ask you to make extra prenatal visits or attend special clinics. You may need to stay in the hospital or to monitor your condition yourself at home. Your doctor my work with a team of experts to provide any special care you may need.

High Blood Pressure

Hypertension, or high blood pressure, occurs when the pressure of the blood in the arteries reaches levels that are greater than normal. This condition can be pre-existing (before pregnancy) and chronic (long-term), or it can arise during pregnancy. High blood pressure that arises during pregnancy can be a sign of a condition called ***preeclampsia*** (also known as toxemia). These two conditions—chronic high blood pressure and preeclampsia—affect pregnancy and its outcome in different ways. Depending on how severe these conditions are, both the mother and fetus can be affected.

Measuring Blood Pressure

Blood pressure is checked with a stethoscope and an instrument made of an inflatable cuff and a pressure gauge (sphygmomanometer). A blood pressure reading is made up of two numbers separated by a slash, for example, 110/80. (You may hear this referred to as "110 over 80.") The first number is the pressure in the arteries when the heart contracts. This is called the systolic pressure. The second number is the pressure in the arteries when the heart is relaxed between contractions. This is the diastolic pressure.

Blood pressure changes often during the day. It can rise if you are excited or if you exercise. It usually falls when you are resting. These temporary changes in blood pressure that occur in response to some activity or event are normal. It is only when a person's blood pressure stays high for some time that it requires attention.

Because of the normal ups and downs in blood pressure, if your doctor finds one high reading, he or she will want to see whether it is your normal level by taking another reading. Your normal blood pressure can be an average of several readings taken at rest.

Blood pressure varies from person to person, so everyone's blood pressure is different. In nonpregnant adults, readings less than 130/80 are usually normal, become abnormal when pressures reach above 140/90.

Some blood pressure levels that may seem normal could be too high in a pregnant woman. For instance, a reading of 120/85 would be considered too high for a pregnant woman whose normal reading was 90/70. As a rule, any increase of 30 or more in the systolic reading or 15 or more in the diastolic reading can be a sign of high blood pressure in pregnancy.

It is normal for blood pressure to drop slightly during the middle part of pregnancy and then return to prepregnancy levels during the latter part of pregnancy. Because of these changes, it is important to have your blood pressure measured before pregnancy or in early pregnancy so your doctor will know what is normal for you. As a part of prenatal care, a woman's blood pressure is checked at each visit.

Warning Signs and Symptoms of High Blood Pressure

These signs and symptoms are sometimes linked to high blood pressure in pregnancy and should warn you to have your blood pressure checked:

- Severe and constant headaches
- Swelling (*edema*), especially of the face
- Dizziness

- Blurred vision or spots in front of the eyes
- Sudden weight gain of more than about 1 pound a day

Chronic High Blood Pressure

High blood pressure can be present when a woman becomes pregnant. Diet, life style, and heredity contribute to chronic high blood pressure. Over the course of her life, a woman with untreated high blood pressure is more likely to have a heart attack or stroke. She is also at higher risk for having problems during pregnancy. These include having a baby that is too small or separation of the ***placenta*** from the wall of the uterus before the fetus is born.

Before you get pregnant, chronic hypertension should be brought under control with diet, weight loss, and possibly medication. During pregnancy, regular checkups are important to detect any changes in your condition that may signal a problem.

Preeclampsia

High blood pressure that occurs for the first time in the second half of pregnancy along with protein in the urine and, usually, fluid retention is called preeclampsia. It affects about 7 out of every 100 women who become pregnant. It is not known what causes preeclampsia, although women who have chronic high blood pressure are more likely to develop it. Most women with preeclampsia, however, have never had high blood pressure before. Preeclampsia usually occurs with first pregnancies and often does not recur in later pregnancies except in women who have chronic hypertension or other diseases affecting the blood vessels. With preeclampsia, blood pressure returns to normal levels after pregnancy, whereas chronic hypertension remains after delivery.

The blood vessels in the uterus supply blood to the placenta, through which the fetus in nourish and given oxygen. When a woman has preeclampsia, the blood flow through these vessels is reduced. The severity of the condition and the time in pregnancy when it occurs determines the degree of risk to the fetus.

When blood pressure increases during pregnancy, your doctor may recommend bed rest. Frequently, the blood pressure will improve or return to normal with rest. When resting, the woman may be advised to lie on her side—this position improves the flow of blood to the uterus and kidneys. Some doctors hospitalize women as soon as there is a slight increase in blood pressure; others wait until there is evidence that bed rest at home has not helped to reduce blood pressure.

Preeclampsia occurs in degrees, from mild to severe, and can gradually worsen or improve. If preeclampsia is detected in mild stages and controlled by bed rest and medication, the effects on the baby can be reduced. The goal, all other factors permitting, is to allow the pregnancy to continue until the fetus is old enough to be born.

When preeclampsia occurs early and is severe, early delivery may be necessary. A premature baby is underweight and may have trouble breathing because the lungs are not fully developed. When preeclampsia is associated with chronic hypertension, the placenta can separate from the uterus and result in ***stillbirth.*** Preeclampsia can also be linked to poor fetal growth. Severe preeclampsia can be fatal to the mother, although this is very rare. The disease affects almost all of the mother's organs, such as the blood system, liver, kidneys, and brain. Convulsions can occur without warning with preeclampsia. When this occurs, the disease is called eclampsia. The treatment for very severe preeclampsia or eclampsia is to deliver the fetus, either by inducing labor or performing a cesarean birth.

Diabetes

diabetes is a condition that occurs when there is a problem with the way the body makes or uses ***insulin.*** Insulin is a hormone that helps the body use ***glucose,*** a sugar that is the body's main source of fuel. When the body doesn't make enough insulin, or when the usual effect of insulin or glucose does not occur as it should, the level of glucose in the blood becomes too high because it is not being used by the body properly. Diabetes can be present before pregnancy or develop during pregnancy. With either type, insulin may be needed to control glucose levels.

Gestational Diabetes

Some women develop diabetes when they become pregnant. This is called gestational diabetes. It results from the effects of hormones made by the placenta during pregnancy. These hormones can alter the way in which insulin works. When abnormal glucose levels first develop during pregnancy, they can do so without symptoms. Usually, the glucose level returns to normal after delivery. Women who have gestational diabetes have a higher risk of developing diabetes again later in life, however.

Diabetes is more likely to occur during pregnancy in women who are age 30 and older, obese, have had problems such as stillbirth or a very large baby in a previous pregnancy, and have a family history of diabetes. If one or more of these risk factors exist, your doctor may decide to test you for diabetes during pregnancy. This safe and simple test is usually done about two-thirds of the way through your pregnancy. A sample of blood is taken exactly 1 hour after you drink a special sugar solution. If the blood glucose level is high, a similar but longer test, usually taking 3 hours, will be done. This is called a glucose tolerance test.

Women who have uncomplicated gestational diabetes may not need insulin; instead, they can control their blood glucose levels by eating a special diet. In this case, blood glucose levels usually are not tested daily. When insulin is used to control gestational diabetes, the diet and the insulin dose must be regulated to prevent the harmful effects of high and low blood glucose levels.

If risks are not controlled, the risk of having a large baby (***macrosomia***) increases. Large babies have difficulty at birth, particularly in delivery of the shoulders. Special testing may be necessary to evaluate the fetus before it is born.

With gestational diabetes, blood glucose levels usually return to normal after birth, but diabetes can recur. You may have another test several months after delivery to make sure you are no longer diabetic. If you are overweight, you and your doctor will set up a balanced program of diet and exercise for you to follow after delivery. This may reduce the risk of problems in later pregnancies and may help lower the risk of developing diabetes later in life.

Preexisting Diabetes

About 1% of women of childbearing age have diabetes. At one time, diabetes posed a major health risk to the mother and fetus during pregnancy. Today, however, more is known about diabetes and how to control it, so pregnancy is safer for most diabetic women.

The outlook for diabetic pregnancies gets better each day. It has improved to the point where the risks for a diabetic pregnancy are almost as low as those for a normal uncomplicated pregnancy. The degree of risk posed by diabetes is directly related to how well the condition is controlled before and during pregnancy. Ideally, the diabetes should be diagnosed and brought under control before pregnancy, and then carefully monitored to keep blood glucose levels as normal as possible. With careful planning, control of diabetes, and expert care, the chances for a successful pregnancy—a healthy baby and mother—are very good.

Risks. although there is no cure for diabetes, it can be effectively treated, and there is less risk to the fetus when the condition is under control before and during pregnancy. Woman who have diabetes when they become pregnant should receive early care to help lower these risks:

- Preeclampsia, or high blood pressure during pregnancy, can require the baby to be delivered early or can slow its growth while in the uterus.
- ***Hydramnios*** (too much ***amniotic fluid*** in the sac surrounding the fetus) can make it difficult for the mother to breathe and may also result in premature labor and delivery.

- Macrosomia (a larger-than-normal baby) occurs in less severe cases and can make delivery difficult.
- Birth defects are more common in babies of diabetic mothers, especially if the diabetes is not well controlled.
- *Miscarriage* occurs more often in diabetic women, especially if the condition is not under control.
- *Respiratory distress syndrome* may affect the baby's ability to breathe because the lungs are not fully developed.
- Stillbirth, although uncommon, also occurs more often in babies of diabetic mothers.

Controlling Diabetes. Your diet is an important way to control your glucose levels. The number of calories in your diet will depend on both your weight and the stage of pregnancy. Your doctor may adjust your diet from time to time to improve blood glucose control or to meet the needs of the growing fetus. Usually the diet consists of special meals and snacks spread throughout the day. A bedtime snack helps to maintain blood glucose levels during the night.

Regular exercise also plays an important role in the control of diabetes. It reduces the amount of insulin needed to maintain normal blood glucose levels. The amount of exercise that is right for each woman varies. Among other things, it depends on the stage of pregnancy.

Some diabetics need to take insulin to keep their blood glucose at a normal level. Insulin can be taken by injection only. It does not cross the placenta, so it does not affect the fetus directly. The amount of insulin needed to control blood glucose levels throughout the day varies from woman to woman and depends on many factor. In many cases, insulin must be taken at least twice a day during pregnancy. Usually the need for insulin increases throughout the pregnancy, leveling off near the end. This means that the insulin dose needs to be adjusted from time to time for good control of blood glucose levels. This is where home monitoring of blood glucose levels plays an important role.

If you have diabetes that must be controlled with insulin, you will need to monitor your blood glucose on a day-to-day basis to keep it at a normal level as much of the time as possible. There are a number of ways to do this, all of which are safe and simple to use. You and your doctor will decide together on the best method or combination of methods for you.

Blood glucose meters or colored strips can be used to measure blood glucose levels at home. In either method, a simple device is used to obtain a small drop of blood, usually from the tip of the finger The blood glucose level is then read with the meter or strip. Both of these methods provide reliable results when used properly.

Because the blood glucose level normally changes throughout the day, it usually must be checked several times a day. Your doctor will advise you as to how often you will need to check you blood glucose.

When diabetes is not controlled and the body cannot use glucose for energy, it resorts to burning fat. Certain substances called ketones produced as a result of burning the fat may be found in the urine. Ketones in the urine can be a sign of ketoacidosis, a serious complication of uncontrolled diabetes that can cause stillbirth.

Special Care for Diabetics. A woman with diabetes usually needs to have certain tests done more often in her pregnancy. These tests can help the doctor identify problems that may occur early and take steps to correct them. One test measures hemoglobin A1C, a substance in the mother's blood. When levels are higher than normal, they indicate that the control of the body's glucose use has been poor for a number of weeks. Other tests, such as ***ultrasound, amniocentesis,*** and fetal monitoring, are used to assess the present status and growth of the fetus. These tests are especially important if the baby must be delivered early.

Early in your pregnancy, you may need to stay briefly in a hospital so that your blood glucose levels can be controlled and your general health can be assessed. additional hospital stays may be needed, depending on your blood glucose levels and any other health problems you may be having. The trend has been to reduce the length of these hospital stays.

At one time, almost all women with diabetes had cesarean births because the potential problems associated with diabetic pregnancy could be made worse by the added stress of labor and vaginal delivery. Today, however, with special tests and monitoring methods, most women with diabetes are able to give birth safely through the vagina.

Heart Disease

Women who have heart disease during their reproductive years may have either rheumatic heart disease or congenital heart disease. Because of advances in preventing rheumatic heart disease, it is a less common problem in pregnancy. Women with congenital heart disease are born with an anatomic defect in the heart. The nature and severity of this defect determine whether they may be at risk of having problems during pregnancy.

Ideally, heart disease should be diagnosed before conception. Once the condition is diagnosed, all possible steps can be taken to correct it. Counseling also can be provided about the impact of the disease on the pregnancy and vice versa. If you have serious cardiac disease, your doctor will work in a team approach with a cardiologist to manage your care throughout the pregnancy.

Pregnancy increases the work the heart has to do, and labor and delivery place added stress on the heart. The amount of blood the heart pumps increases by up to 40% during pregnancy. Physical activity may need to be limited so that the demand on the heart is lessened. Your doctor will prescribe a routine of rest and possibly medications.

During labor, contractions increase the heart's work load, as do the pain and anxiety that go along with them. In spite of this, when obstetric conditions permit, vaginal delivery is preferred over cesarean birth because it causes less stress to the heart. ***Anesthesia*** may be given during labor to reduce pain and anxiety.

Women with heart disease are more likely to deliver prematurely, and their babies are often smaller than they should be. The babies of mothers who have congenital heart disease have a 4–5% chance of having the disease as well, although it may not be serious or life-threatening. New techniques for diagnosing heart disease in the fetus have improved the accuracy of this diagnosis and make it possible to plan for special care.

Lung Disorders

pregnancy causes a number of changes in a woman's breathing patterns. Due to the growing uterus, the shape of the chest cavity is changed. It is quite common for a pregnant woman to feel short of breath (for hints on ways to feel more comfortable when you are short of breath, There are certain lung disorders, however, that may cause changes beyond this common shortness of breath.

Asthma, a lung disorder that causes wheezing and breathing problems, is one of the more common problems. It has not been shown to worsen or improve during pregnancy, but it could pose problems if the fetus does not get enough oxygen. Most women with asthma can go safely through a pregnancy, continuing to use their inhalers or prescribed medicines to help them breathe and supply the fetus with enough oxygen. Most of the medicines used for asthma are safe during pregnancy, except those containing iodine or tetracycline. Therefore, your doctor needs to know which medicines you take. Women with severe asthma must have their problem carefully controlled and be watched closely, because their asthma attacks will probably continue during pregnancy.

Pneumonia is an infection in the lungs that may be more serious in pregnancy than it is at other times. It may result in the mother and fetus getting less oxygen, and so it should be diagnosed and treated promptly. A chest X-ray is usually an important step in finding pneumonia. The technician who takes the X-ray may place a lead apron on your abdomen to shield the fetus. This type of X-ray has not been shown to cause any harm to the fetus. A pregnant woman with pneumonia is often hospitalized to receive ***antibiotics,*** many of which are safe for the mother and fetus.

Renal Disease

During pregnancy, more blood flows to the kidneys as they work harder to filter waste products faster to take care of the needs of both the woman and her fetus. If a woman's kidneys are weakened from a previous disease or do not work properly, it could have an effect on her pregnancy. With proper medical treatment, however, risks usually can be reduced. Some disorders that affect the kidney are linked with high blood pressure. If the blood pressure can be controlled, the risk of problems during pregnancy is reduced.

Kidney disease can usually be diagnosed on the basis of your medical history, physical exam, and blood and urine tests. Protein in the urine may be a sign of kidney disease. It can be caused by diseases that interfere with kidney function. Urinary tract infections and high blood pressure in a previous pregnancy also are signs that require further evaluation.

Epilepsy

Women with epilepsy or seizures (convulsions) can have safe pregnancies. Seizures may be minor problems involving muscle control or major attacks involving loss of control of bladder or bowel function and blackout spells. Usually women with seizures take medicines prescribed to control or prevent repeated seizures.

A woman with epilepsy has a risk two to three times higher than normal of having a baby with a birth defect, especially cleft lip and palate or heart defects. The reason for the higher risk is not clear. It is known, however, that some of the drugs taken to control seizures can cause birth defects. However, a seizure or repeated seizures could be harmful to the mother or fetus as well. Therefore, a woman with epilepsy should discuss continued drug use with her doctor. Sometimes the medication can be changed before or during pregnancy to reduce the risks.

Autoimmune Disorders

The autoimmune disorders are a group of diseases in which the body's immune system, which is designed to protect it, goes awry, attacking and injuring the body's own tissues. The injury may be in a specific organ, such as the kidney, or in various parts of the body.

Most autoimmune diseases are chronic conditions for which there is no cure. It is not always known what causes them. Their symptoms can disappear for a time and then recur with little warning or without apparent reason. The effects on pregnancy depend on the type of disorder.

Many of the autoimmune diseases have overlapping signs and symptoms, making them difficult to diagnose. your doctor may work with a specialist in planning care for your pregnancy.

Systemic Lupus Erythematosus

Systemic lupus erythematosus (SLE) is a disease that can affect the entire body, including skin, joints, kidneys, and the nervous system. Its results can range from minor skin sores to a serious fatal condition in which the kidneys fail and the nervous system, heart, and blood are affected.

SLE tends to occur in young women during their childbearing years. It does not appear to affect fertility, but it increases the risks of miscarriage, premature deliveries, and stillbirth. A baby of a woman with SLE can be born with a heart defect.

In approximately 30% of women with SLE, the disease becomes more severe during pregnancy, and symptoms can worsen after delivery. If the disease is in remission 6 months before conception and the woman's kidneys are not involved, the chances of having a healthy baby are considered good.

SLE is treated with drugs called corticosteroids. There is no evidence that these drugs are harmful to the fetus. Your doctor may also prescribe aspirin and aspirin-like drugs to control joint pain. Usually the dosage is kept as low as possible during pregnancy to avoid effects such as fetal bleeding.

Rheumatoid Arthritis

Rheumatoid arthritis is thought of as a disease of the joints because it most often causes inflammation, pain, tenderness, heat, and swelling, particularly of the small and medium-sized joints. It is accompanied by morning stiffness and a general feeling of fatigue and discomfort. The condition can flare up and then lessen for a time, or it can become worse and worse, damaging joints. In addition, rheumatoid arthritis can affect the blood—resulting in severe anemia—or other systems of the body.

Many women find that their rheumatoid arthritis improves during pregnancy, although some have a relapse between 6 weeks and 6 months after delivery. Rheumatoid arthritis can be treated with aspirin-like drugs and sometimes other drugs during pregnancy.

Thyroid Disease

The thyroid gland can be affected by diseases that cause it to be overactive or underactive. Either can have harmful effects of the fetus. Hypothyroidism, or an underactive condition, is treated with thyroid hormone pills. Blood tests are used to determine whether the amount of hormone being taken is sufficient.

Medicines also are available to treat hyperthy-roidism, or an overactive thyroid gland. The proper dose of these medicines is determined by blood tests. A patient with thyroid disease that is properly controlled during pregnancy can have a normal pregnancy.

What You Can Do

If you have a chronic disease, it is best to see your doctor before you become pregnant. If this is not possible, make an appointment as soon as you know you are pregnant. You have probably already worked out a routine for control and treatment with your family doctor or a specialist. Now your routine may need to be changed. You may have to adjust medication schedules, types, and doses to accommodate your pregnancy. If your condition is well controlled during pregnancy, your efforts will be rewarded by improving the chance of having a healthy baby.

If you are just learning now that you have some sort of illness, it can come as a shock. On top of learning about pregnancy and delivery, you must learn how to care for a medical condition. Your doctor or a specialist that your doctor recommends can help you adjust and work out a course of treatment. Pregnancy can affect medical conditions in many ways, and you may find that your condition is better after you deliver your baby.

The best actions you can take to increase the chances of having a healthy baby are to keep your condition under control, to see your doctor regularly, and to follow his or her instructions. Having a chronic medical condition that needs treatment does complicate your pregnancy, but most women with these conditions have healthy babies. You can, too.

Questions to Consider....

- Since I have a medical condition before pregnancy, should the doctor who is treating that condition be consulted?
- Is it all right to continue to take medication prescribed before I became pregnant?
- If I have high blood pressure, will it return to normal after the baby is born?

- If I have gestational diabetes, what can I do to keep it from returning later?
- How often will my condition need to be evaluated during my pregnancy?